Praise for *The Art of Plant-Based Cheesemaking*

Karen brings an enormous wealth of knowledge and experience to the world of plant-based cheese making. Her innovative techniques that honor time-tested tradition will inform the future of dairy-free food products. Having had the opportunity to taste many Blue Heron Creamery cheeses, it is clear that under Karen's lead, a revolution in dairy freedom has been sparked.

MARGARET COONS founder and CEO, Nuts for Cheese

More than a compilation of recipes, *The Art of Plant-Based Cheesemaking* is an in-depth course for every would-be cheese crafter and culinary artisan. With luscious, full-color photos of finished cheeses and step-by-step instructions replete with visual aids, McAthy deconstructs the cheesemaking process to make it accessible to everybody. From quick non-cultured cheezes to fresh and aged cultured cheeses, no curd is left behind. Think it's impossible to go vegan because you can't live without cheese? Think again! This book will quash all your excuses.

JO STEPANIAK, MSEd author, *Low-FODMAP and Vegan*, *The Ultimate Uncheese Cookbook*, and *Vegan Vittles*

Delightful, inspiring, and delicious! *The Art of Plant-based Cheesemaking* is alive with possibilities, beauty, and love. This book draws a map for pleasure and exploration, simple and complex—like life.

LAURA CUSHNIE co-founder and Executive Chef, la Dulse Vie

The Art of Plant-Based Cheesemaking is an intimate and academic invitation into the brilliant mind and fermenting-friendly kitchen of Karen McAthy. For the time that I have known Karen, I have always wondered what magic she inserted into her delicious and innovative plant-inspired food. From the first time I tried her cheeze at Graze to the incredible pate that she included in my book launch, I am filled with intense excitement at the opportunity to take her mind into my kitchen and create these evolutionary products. Karen has created an approachable and researched method for both vegans and non-vegans to appreciate and enjoy this lifestyle with ease and confidence.

CHLOE ELGAR holistic nutritionist and author
and founder, Chloe's Countertop

Once upon a time cheese was the stumbling block for many on the path to a plant-based diet. Plant-based cheeses were both unhealthful and unpalatable. The tide has turned. *The Art of Plant-Based Cheesemaking* is destined to be a classic that propels plant-based cheesemaking to the next level. For everyone who ever wanted to knock someone's socks off with non-dairy cheese, this book is your ticket to success. It is a beautiful compilation of exquisite recipes masterfully crafted by Karen McAthy. We are both awed and grateful!

BRENDA DAVIS AND VESANTO MELINA registered dietitians
and co-authors, *Becoming Vegan: Comprehensive Edition*,
www.becomingvegan.ca

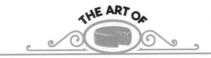

THE ART OF

PLANT-BASED CHEESEMAKING

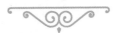

how to craft real, cultured,
- non-dairy cheese -

KAREN McATHY

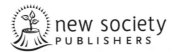

new society
PUBLISHERS

Cover design by Diane McIntosh. Cover photo © Catherine Downes
Interior design by Setareh Ashrafologhalai.

Printed in Canada. First printing March 2017.

Inquiries regarding requests to reprint all or part of *The Art of Plant-Based Cheesemaking* should be addressed to New Society Publishers at the address below. To order directly from the publishers, please call toll-free (North America) 1-800-567-6772, or order online at www.newsociety.com

Any other inquiries can be directed by mail to:
New Society Publishers
P.O. Box 189, Gabriola Island, BC V0R 1X0, Canada
(250) 247-9737

LIBRARY AND ARCHIVES CANADA CATALOGUING IN PUBLICATION

McAthy, Karen, author
    The art of plant-based cheesemaking : how to craft real, cultured, non-dairy cheese / Karen McAthy.

Issued in print and electronic formats.
ISBN 978-0-86571-836-4 (softcover).--ISBN 978-1-55092-631-6 (PDF).
--ISBN 978-1-77142-225-3 (HTML)

    1. Milk-free diet--Recipes. 2. Dairy substitutes. 3. Cheesemaking--Handbooks, manuals, etc. 4. Vegan cooking. 5. Cheese. 6. Cookbooks.
I. Title.

RM234.5.M37 2017   641.5'63   C2017-901006-9   C2017-901007-7

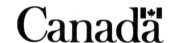

| Funded by the Government of Canada | Financé par le gouvernement du Canada |

New Society Publishers' mission is to publish books that contribute in fundamental ways to building an ecologically sustainable and just society, and to do so with the least possible impact on the environment, in a manner that models this vision.

▶ Blue Heron Creamery cheeses. CATHERINE DOWNES

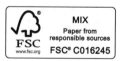

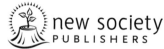

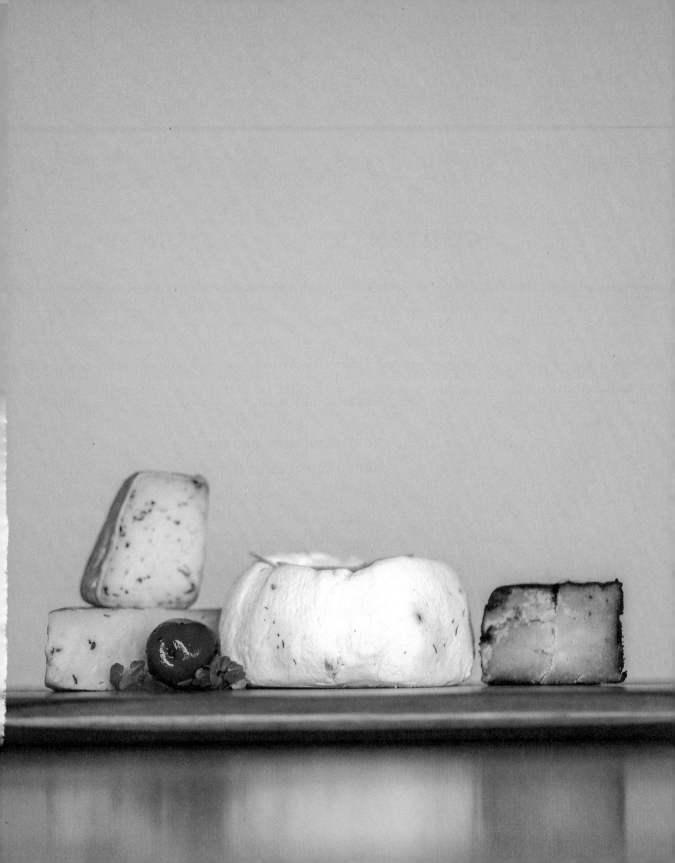

CONTENTS

ACKNOWLEDGMENTS

GETTING TO THIS book has been such an incredible journey. I like to make things. I like to understand how things work. I like to learn new things. I never thought I would write a book and certainly never intended to. I have had the great fortune to be surrounded by many people who have supported and actively encouraged my pursuits, and I am ever grateful to them as I continue this perpetual journey of learning. I am humbled that somehow this has led to a book, and to my company, Blue Heron Creamery.

This book would not have happened without them.

I am forever grateful to all of the clients and guests who have eaten my food and my cheeses and keep wanting to — I know some of you by name and am fortunate to have met too many of you to name individually here.

Michael Lyons — Graze Vegetarian was such an incredible experience to be part of, all of it.

Eden Chan — such an incredible experience to continue our creative culinary journey together, thank you.

Aaron Leung, James Davison, Laura Cushnie — the sous chefs who tolerated me, grew with me, and did not hesitate every time I wanted to experiment with something, gave me pause, and taught me many things, and with whom I still confer.

Jess Borthwick, Sam Tong, Amber Meredith, Lori McIntosh — for so many reasons (too many to list), but to have worked with you all, and to know you all, I am grateful that you have been a part of so many important things along the way.

Katie Luebke — I look forward to an opportunity to work alongside you again, you were the right person at the right time.

Zoe Peled, Colin Medhurst, Catherine Downes — for being such an important part of Blue Heron's birth and continued evolution.

Ryan Lanji — because, everything.

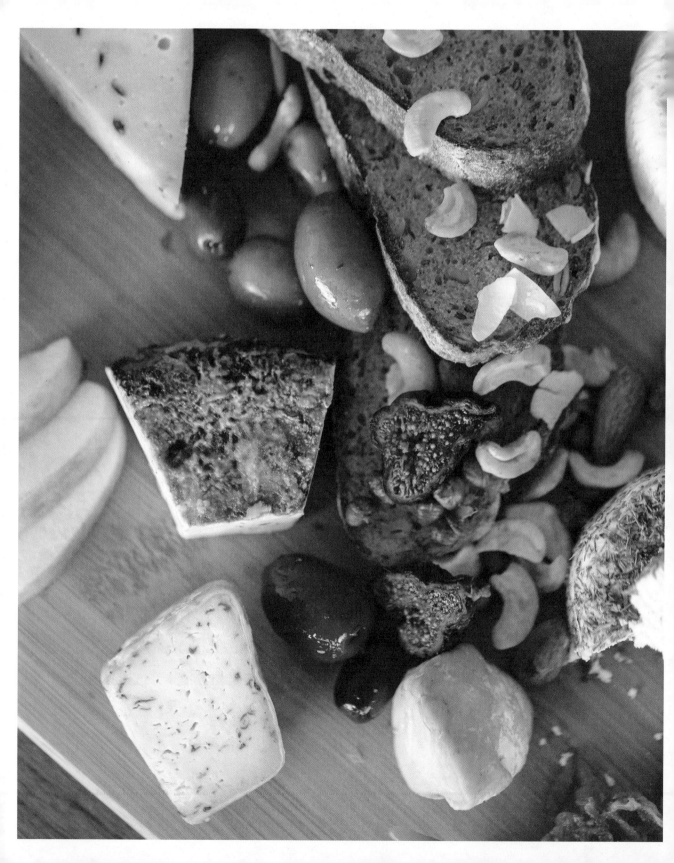

FOREWORD

IN THE SPRING of 2013 I accepted the post as Executive Chef of Graze Vegetarian, a new, plant-based restaurant Michael Lyons was opening in Vancouver, B.C. Creating a solely plant-based menu that would have broad appeal and yet be creatively interesting was our primary goal. As part of that, we decided plant-based, dairy-free cheese, or cheese analog, would have a place on the menu.

Wanting to offer something that was more in line with traditional cheesemaking, and therefore cultured and aged, I began exploring beyond the plentiful cheeze recipes and processes. Certainly, I did (and do) make some offerings that fell fully within that realm, but I wanted to understand the culturing and aging process more deeply, and began experimenting with different cultures, different combination of nuts, seeds, even legumes, and different aging and curing methods.

The initial cultured cheeses, were primarily in either the "ricotta" or "chevre" style and employed rejuvelac (see Chapter 4), sauerkraut brine, or probiotic capsules. The results, while interesting, and able to create tasty cheese-like results, always seemed limited to one note with respect to acidity and flavor. As I began to think more about what cheesemaking itself is, I was fortunate enough to have a young woman, Katie Luebke, apply to stage with me at Graze.

◀ Blue Heron Creamery cheese board. CATHERINE DOWNES

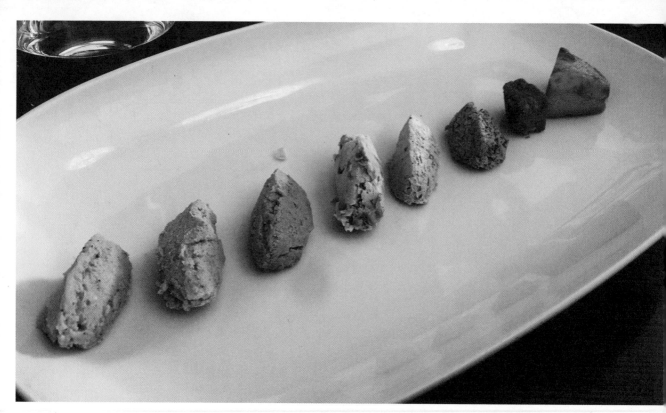

▲ Graze Vegetarian cheese test samples. AUTHOR

Katie, already working full time as a cook at another restaurant, had heard that I was doing a lot of fermentation and culturing and making plant-based cheeses. She had a serious interest in culturing processes herself, and spent two days a week for nearly six months in the Graze kitchen, helping me carry out a variety of experiments, testing mediums, cultures, aging processes, archiving the cheese and taking notes — so many notes.

As we explored the limitations of rejuvelac culturing to create depth of flavour in plant-based cheeses, I began researching traditional (dairy) cheesemaking methods and cultures in an attempt to identify what makes cheese ... well, cheese.

In the course of reading and researching, I began thinking of cheese as a concept. I also began thinking of it as the end outcome of several processes relying on the application of cultures (mold, fungi,

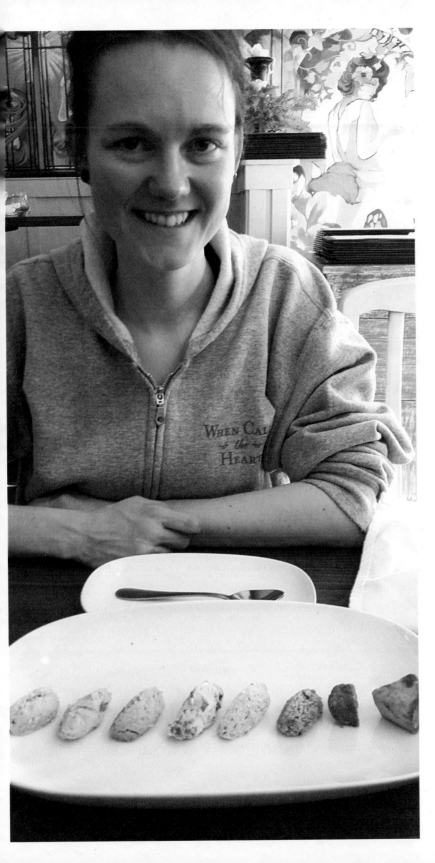

◀ Katie at Graze with cheese samples. AUTHOR

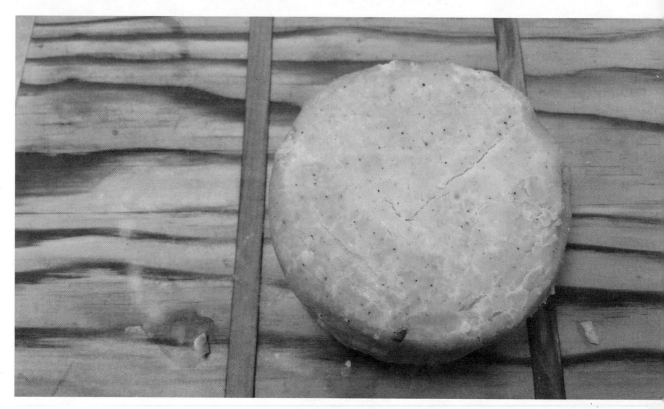

▲ Cheese at Graze. AUTHOR

yeast, bacteria) on a medium (traditionally, animal dairy) and, in many cases, aged and cured through the application of other processes such as air-drying, salt brining, washing rinds with wine, wax aging, and so on. Thinking in this way allowed me to consider the various steps as discrete, and then to understand that the medium upon which cultures were applied could, at least in theory, be changed from dairy to plant-based.

This conceptualization is what ultimately invigorated my desire to test and refine my own plant-based cheesemaking approach, and indeed informs what I understand cheese to be.

After Katie and I began pursuing this understanding through further tests, we had a number of happy surprises, a few unexpected results, and, of course, some things that didn't quite work out as desired. Our effort resulted in being able to sell some of the cheeses at the Vancouver Farmers Markets in 2015. After the closure

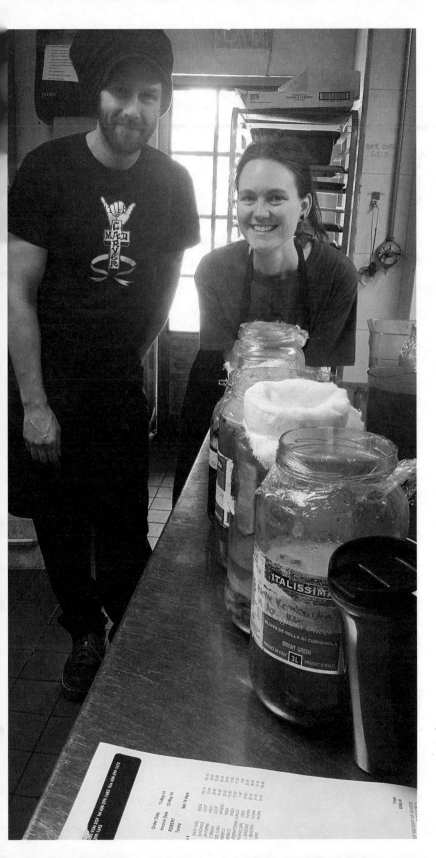

◀ Jamie and Katie, Mother's Day at Graze. AUTHOR

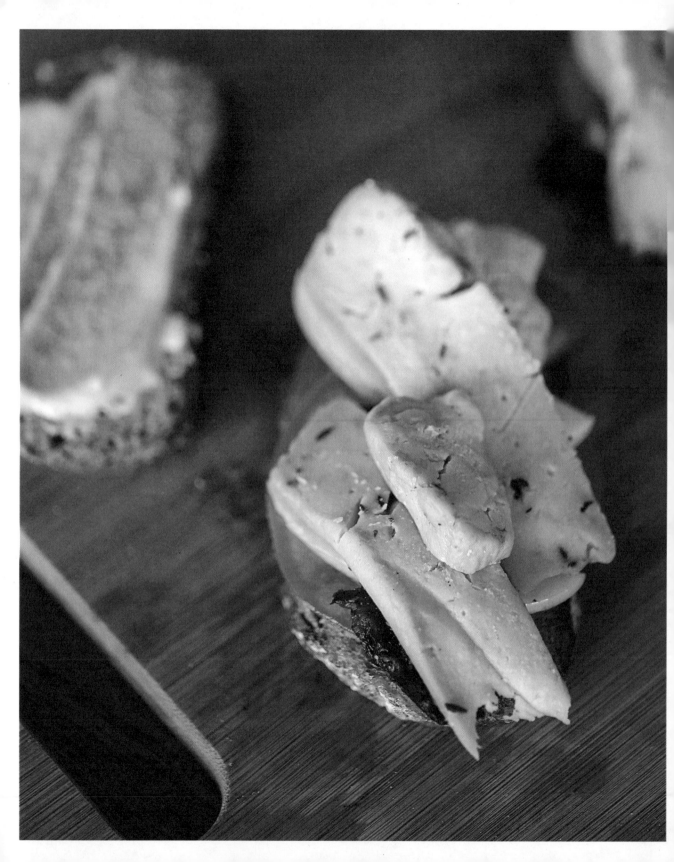

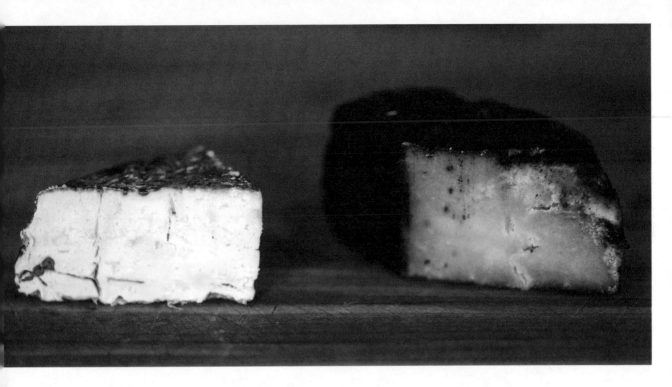

of Graze Vegetarian in November 2015, I continued to develop the processes I use and the cheeses I make and launched Blue Heron Cheese (plant-based, dairy-free) in April 2016.

Of all the things I've learned, the most important is that this is an exploration driven by endless curiosity, and that I myself am a novice. Making cheese and working with cultures mean learning constantly, developing patience, and studying the smallest details — something I hope to be doing for a very long time.

This book is an invitation to the seriously interested cheese-maker to participate with me in an exploration and development of cheese. To choose patience, observation, and time over speed and instant gratitude.

It is an invitation to deeper understanding and, therefore, more care. More care about making food. More care about where food comes from. More care about how we feed ourselves and share with others. Making food, and cheese, is ultimately the way I choose to express love.

◀ Blue Heron Creamery cheese — Caraway Gouda on rye. CATHERINE DOWNES

▲ Almond coconut blue and balsamic vinegar-washed aged blue. CATHERINE DOWNES

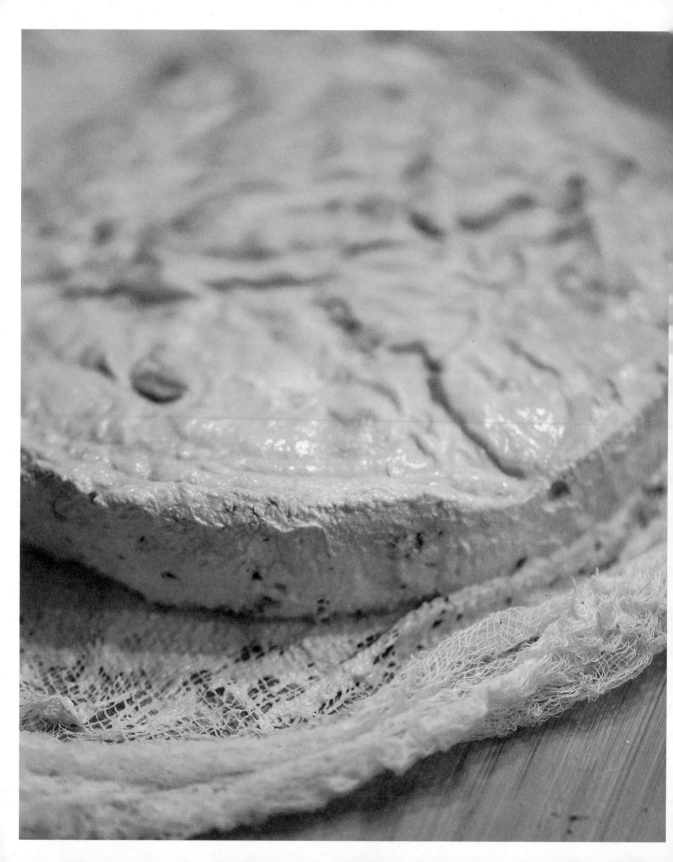

INTRODUCTION

CHEESE. CREAMY, SHARP, firm, tangy, pungent — the sensory adjectives are plentiful. The redolent textures and aromas of this cultured food have inspired many a romantic obsession. There are thousands of varieties of cheese, all cultured from goat's milk, cow's milk, sheep's milk, and even buffalo's milk. In principle it is a simple food. Rarely made up of more than four to five ingredients — a medium (animal milk), salt, enzymes, microbial cultures, a coagulating agent — cheese maintains an almost primitive hold on the human palette.

Cheese is one of the oldest of modern foods. Humans across nearly every culture have developed some form of animal milk into this cultured and aged foodstuff that has grown from a humble survival food eaten by peasants to high end, artisan craft. An accident of circumstance (lack of refrigeration for preserving milk) and organisms (bacteria and molds), cheese is a by-product of fermentation, culturing, and time (aging).

Like all forms of fermentation and culturing, cheesemaking evolved as a means of preserving food for the long months after the harvest when food was sparse. Now, along with many fermented and cultured food practices, such as sauerkraut, kimchi, tempeh, beer and wine, cheesemaking has become one of a growing number of

◀ Blue Heron Creamery Black Trumpet Mushroom Cashew Camembert. CATHERINE DOWNES

do-it-yourself pursuits of ardent foodies. In recent years, a number of books have been written with this pursuit in mind, including *The Cheesemaker's Apprentice* by Sasha Davies and *Mastering Basic Cheesemaking* by Gianaclis Caldwell. Cheesemaking kits, with the home user in mind, are readily available either online or in boutique food shops, allowing people to explore making their own ricotta, cream cheese, burrata, mozzarella, and others.

Cheese, and cheesemaking, are inherently involved in an ongoing evolution, and the latest area of development is the pursuit of plant-based, dairy-free alternatives. Understanding why this pursuit has gained traction is relevant. As plant-based and vegan eating and lifestyle choices in general have moved from the periphery of most cultures to the mainstream of many, especially in some of North America and Western Europe, forsaking cheese is often seen as the last barrier to overcome.

Three core areas of concern inform the embracing of plant-based/plant-forward eating and lifestyle choices, particularly in the West: environmental, personal health and animal welfare. As evidence mounts for the benefits of, at the very least, minimizing as much as possible our consumption of animal products for both personal health and environmental reasons, a growing market is seeking alternatives to favorite items. This has included a surge in alternatives to cheese.

One of the most significant evolutions in cheesemaking in recent years has been the pursuit of plant-based cheesemaking. In many ways, Miyoko Schinner's book *Artisan Vegan Cheese* set the stage for this evolution, advancing the idea of plant-based, dairy-free cheese beyond cheesy flavored pâtés and spreads, which have primarily filled the void for those avoiding dairy cheese. Putting forward recipes that involve some degree of culturing (probiotic application), and flavor outcomes that are at least somewhat familiar, Schinner's book has inspired many home foodie and prospective artisan plant-based cheesemakers alike.

▶ Blue Heron Creamery Herbed Coconut Kefir cheese. CATHERINE DOWNES

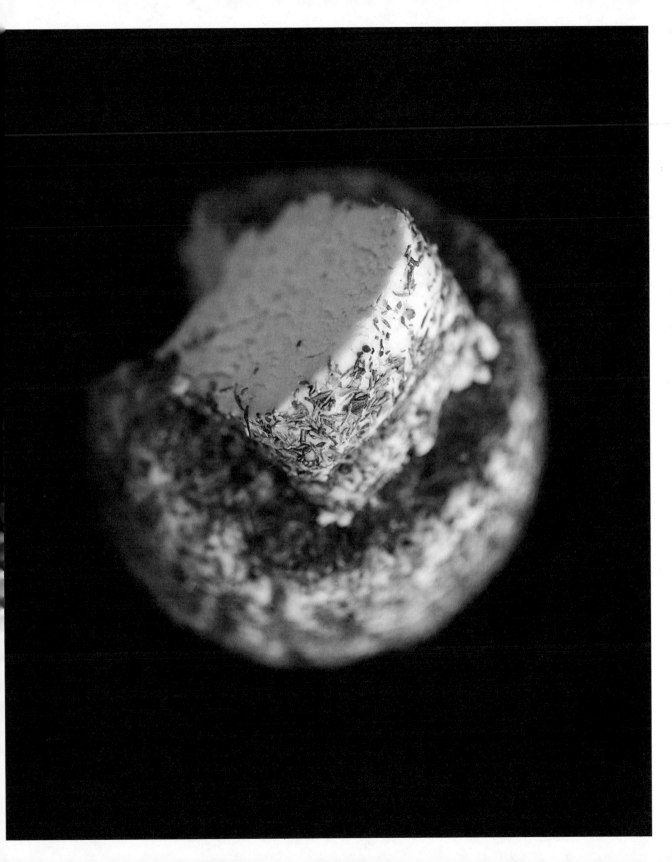

A claim that these processes and recipes constitute some form of cheese is indeed controversial. The United Nations Codex Alimentarius (or Food Code) essentially defines cheese as the product created by the culturing of dairy proteins. The Codex is a set of "... international food standards, guidelines and codes of practice that contribute to the safety, quality, and fairness of [the] international food trade..." For a list of the cheese standards outlined by the Codex, visit fao.org. Many ardent cheese lovers and makers alike would indeed balk at the notion that a plant-based dairy-free cheese could be made and be legitimately understood as cheese.

However, just as there has been an evolution of dairy cheesemaking to include different flavors and now, even, coconut milk, there has been a considerable movement forward in non-dairy cheese processes and products. Many plant-based cheesemakers such as Miyoko Schinner (Miyoko's Kitchen, California), Tal Ronnen (Kite Hill, California), Margaret Coons (Nuts for Cheese, London, Ontario, Canada), Blöde Kuh (California), Cheezehound (New York), Happy Cheeze (Germany), and Blue Heron (Vancouver, British Columbia, Canada) are exploring varying degrees of fermentation and culturing processes in an effort to create products which have more depth, flavor and cheese-like qualities than previous analogs which were primarily flavored starches or other combinations of ingredients, such as compressed plant proteins and seasonings.

Certainly these efforts open the door for those advancing the culturing of non-dairy based mediums. This book sets out to explore the development of plant-based cheeses as a legitimate evolution of cheesemaking itself. It offers a sampling of approaches to plant-based cheeses moving from simpler to more advanced processes, concluding with some elements of my own approach, which seeks to apply, as much as relevant and possible, traditional cheesemaking methods to plant-based mediums.

This book invites the curious reader to try their hand at a few of their own plant-based cheesemaking experiments and to find ways of

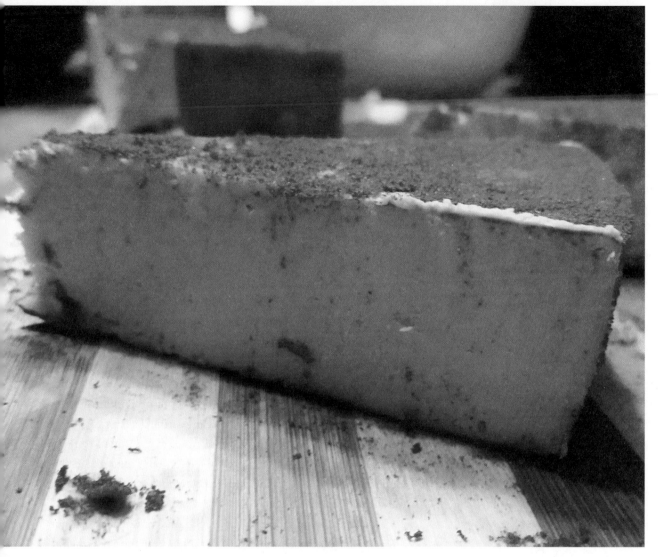

▲ Blue Heron Creamery Smoked Cheddar (cashew). AUTHOR

expanding their personal understanding of what cheese is. As readers explore making and using cultures, they have an opportunity to experiment with creating cheeses to suit their own preferences, to understand how the culturing process works (and sometimes fails), and to become more intimately familiar with a practice that has its roots in hundreds of years of human history and food preservation.

CORE ELEMENTS OF PLANT-BASED CHEESEMAKING

TRADITIONAL CHEESE OR "true cheese" as the New England Cheesemaking Supply Company calls it, is generally defined by the consolidation of milk proteins (casein) with calcium and enzymes (rennet), followed by the development of acidity-using lactic bacteria (lactobacillus) which convert the sugars of the dairy to lactic acid followed by the modification of protein during the aging process, resulting in different textures and flavors.

The Food and Agriculture Organization of the United Nations maintains the Codex Alimentarius, which sets out standardized definitions for food production and identification. The Codex reinforces the above definition.

It does not formally recognize non-animal milk cheese, or nut milks for that matter. However, it is actually within the Codex definition that I find the seed of my own interpretation of cheese.

In the Codex Standard 283–1978, cheese is "... the ripened or unripened soft, semi-hard, or extra-hard product, which may be coated, and in which the whey protein/casein does not exceed that of milk, obtained by:

a. Coagulating wholly or partly the protein of milk, skimmed milk, partly skimmed milk, cream, whey cream or buttermilk, or any combination of these materials, through the action of rennet or other suitable coagulating agents, and by partially draining the whey resulting from the coagulation, while respecting the principle that cheesemaking results in the concentration of milk protein (in particular, the casein portion), and that consequently, the protein content of the cheese will be distinctly higher than the protein level of the blend of the above milk materials from which the cheese was made; and/or

b. Processing techniques involving coagulation of the protein of milk and or products obtained from milk which give an end-product with similar physical, chemical and organoleptic characteristics as the product defined under a)."

It may seem difficult to see how I find my definition of plant-based cheese within these strict confines, but in opening up the traditional and "official" definition of cheese, I am choosing to understand and evaluate cheese as a concept. That is, I have elected to pull apart the Codex definition and focus on its process components: coagulation of protein-rich medium (in my case nut and seed bases), acidification of the medium with a lactic acid culture, and in some cases, modification of proteins through aging processes.

Through experimentation and ongoing study of traditional approaches in cheesemaking, I mirror the true cheese definition in that there are some essential components underlying what constitutes cheese. I use starter cultures, primarily lactic acid cultures, enzymes for coagulation (vegetable rennet where applicable), and potable water. Similar to the true cheese definition, I do not consider the inclusion of thickening agents, oils or emulsifiers as being part of a cheesemaking process. I refer to the products that do use those components as "cheeze." Also, as with true cheese, herbs, fruit, beer/wine can be added.

I do not expect to unravel all of the necessary scientific elements of this claim within this book, but I do hope that the definition I provide is helpful for the reader in understanding how I define cheese and therefore the approach I am taking. It would take considerable

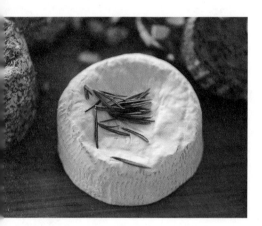

▲ Traditional cheese (dairy) —
Salt Spring Island Cheese
Company brie. CATHERINE DOWNES

scientific testing and evaluation to truly have an impact on rede-fining cheese from the current established view, and that is not the purpose of this book.

Instead I invite the home cheesemaker, plant-based or not, to reconsider the possibilities of cheese, to think outside the confines of its formal definition and to allow the progress of my recipes and methods to reveal the possibility that advanced plant-based cheesemaking could indeed be understood as an evolution of the cheesemaking process itself.

Additionally, in presenting recipes, I also seek to provide a quasi-historical overview of plant-based cheese methods and styles. While not exhaustive, it will give you a good range to choose from for your own home-based experimenting fun.

Making traditional cheese, or true cheese as the New England Cheesemaking Supply Company calls it, confines itself to minimal ingredients, relying on time and conditions such as temperature and humidity, and techniques such as rind-washing, surface culturing, and so forth to create the depth and complexity of flavor and texture. While some cheeses will include elements such as herbs, garlic, wine, beer, and fruit, these are in addition to the primary action of cultur-ing the dairy. Very few dairy cheeses are single-day processes.

In contrast to the long history of dairy-based cheesemaking, like so many of humankind's food preserving methods started out as a bit of an accident, plant-based cheesemaking began with intention. As cheese is often the last hurdle for those desiring to pursue a fully plant-based lifestyle, it comes as no surprise that many, many people have set about to explore a variety of means of creating the flavor and texture that so many people miss.

It is not the intention of this book to identify a strict history of plant-based cheese, nor to speak as an authority on plant-based cheese as a whole. So much of the plant-based food movement has been done in do-it-yourself situations, with people developing and building knowledge and sharing it at the private level. Until relatively recently (the last 30 years), there has been very little available in the way of "formal" culinary education in this realm, and even less so with respect to culturing and fermentation. This parallels, in many ways, how so much food knowledge has always been shared — in the kitchens and at the tables of people at home among friends and family and within community.

TERMINOLOGY: "CHEESE" VERSUS "CHEEZE"

For the purposes of understanding how I understand "cheese," and how I set about defining it, I will employ an informal set of categories. Dairy cheesemaking has its own nomenclature and classification system largely defined by the process and culture used to make the cheese. Surface ripened, washed rind, cave aged, cheddar, etcetera are all *processes*. Camembert, roqueforti, are *cultures*. Soft, semi-soft, and hard cheeses all have specific characteristics, which are applied to identify cheese styles. In many cases, multiple categories apply to one kind of cheese.

Currently there is no official or formal classification system or common nomenclature for identifying plant-based cheeses, either by style or method. For the purposes of guiding you through this book I will use an informal classification system organized first according to whether the cheese is cultured or not, and second according to either texture or process.

The basic categories I will explore are non-cultured "cheezes," and cultured and aged cheeses. Using the word cheeze will mean that I am referring to recipes that do not use cultures or aging processes. The use of the traditional term cheese will imply that recipes with that term are cultured, aged or otherwise mirror some elements of traditional cheesemaking. The cultured and aged cheeses will range from simple fresh cheeses to more advanced cheeses and processes that bring us closer to bridging the gap between dairy and plant-based cheesemaking. These definitions are my own and are not ubiquitous across plant-based cheesemakers.

NON-CULTURED CHEEZE

Cheese analogs, or cheeze, are not cultured. These cheezes generally aim to capture something of the nostalgic texture, taste, and feel of dairy cheese, but without engaging in culturing or aging processes which do the primary work in the creation of dairy cheeses (after the milk production by the animals themselves, of course). The addition of fruits, nuts, herbs, and flavors is much more common among plant-based cheeze than in the traditional realm; the outcome is sometimes, though not always, somewhere between pâté and cheese. Most importantly, this in no way makes them less appealing or delicious to eat!

Non-cultured cheezes are typically made with a nut, seed, or soy base, nutritional yeast, salt, vinegar or lemon juice, starch, and agar agar or other kind of setting agent for a firmer, slicing cheeze. These cheezes can be heated and then shaped or made as raw preparations (without the agar or other thickening agent). To a small extent they can be air dried to remove moisture, but generally have a shorter shelf life due to the lack of acidity which is produced in the culturing of food.

The now almost ubiquitous term "cashew cheese" is a widespread example of the introduction of the idea of plant-based cheese and cheeze into the mainstream. The term "cashew cheese" has no fixed definition (cultured or non-cultured). However, given that many of the "cashew cheese" recipes available online are not cultured, I consider this to be a cheeze, and an analog. With dozens of recipes existing on the internet for a quick cheese-like substance to be used in ravioli, lasagne, salads, and so on, even non-plant-based chefs occasionally try their hand at some version or other. If the recipes do not call for the inclusion of a culture (rejuvelac, probiotic, or other culturing agent), then the end result is cheeze (non-cultured). Recipes for soft, semi-soft, and firm cheezes (non-cultured) will be detailed further on.

This user-friendly analog is highly adaptable and low risk for the home user. It allows for broad experimentation, and multiple applications from sauces to thicker preparations, and without additional ingredients aside from cashews and filtered water, also serves as a base medium for culturing processes that can be used in some cultured cheeses. I think of this as the gateway plant-based cheeze and with its generally broad appeal, cashew cheese at least allows the skeptic to consider the possibility of non-dairy cheese.

CULTURED CHEESE

With cultured and aged cheeses we begin to explore in more depth the realm and effect of culturing and fermentation. Nuts, seeds, or even legumes are soaked (sometimes wild-fermented), blended into a paste or mylk (milk substitute), and then a culturing agent such as rejuvelac, or a probiotic capsule (with lactic acid bacteria) is added. Some plant-based cheesemakers in this realm are exploring double culturing processes, whereby they apply a first culture for the production of lactic acid, then a secondary culture to develop a more complex flavor. This begins to mirror the practices of some types of traditional cheesemaking. Nuts for Cheese, by Margaret Coons in London, Ontario, is one of these cheesemakers.

Typically, these cheeses are cultured for up to 48 hours, then either a secondary culture is added or they are formed, and perhaps some level of rind washing occurs. Aging does not usually take more than a few weeks, and air drying is one of the most common methods of moisture removal. Each cheesemaker has a process they have modified to suit their objectives of taste and texture.

MORE ON INFORMAL CLASSIFICATION

The informal classification I will use to organize the recipes is as follows: fresh/soft cheeses, short-term aged cheeses, and long-term aged cheeses. This last category will present a couple of recipes and methods associated more closely with dairy-based cheesemaking and thereby illuminate the idea that plant-based cheesemaking, at least to some extent, can be considered an evolution of cheesemaking itself.

2

EQUIPMENT, SANITIZATION, AND FOOD SAFETY

FOOD SAFETY AND SANITIZATION

THE IMPORTANCE OF food safety and sanitization cannot be understated when working with cultures. Food safety begins with sanitization, that is, a clean working environment. However, the microbes we are often encouraged to eradicate in the interest of food safety are not always the ones that pose a threat. Cheesemaking inherently involves the use of cultures. "Cultures" is a broad term that includes microbes that humans use to make fermented and cultured foods, such as beer, wine, cheese, yogurt, sour pickles, kombucha, vinegar, kefir, kimchi, sauerkraut and so on. Culturing microbes are yeasts, moulds (members of the fungi family), and bacteria, and they exist everywhere. Many of these microbes are already present on the surface of our skin, in the soil, in the air, on fruits and vegetables, and, importantly, within our digestive systems.

Commercial microbes have been bred and fed on specific mediums and specific strains have been cultivated for use in commercial fermentation (cheesemaking, beer, wine, etc.).

Just as the wild yeast, bacteria, and moulds that we use to culture and ferment food exist everywhere, so do the microbes that we have come to fear (with reason), and have developed much of modern-day food safety and sanitization principles around. Salmonella, botulinum, E. coli, and listeria are among the microbes we are most concerned about with regard to ensuring safe food production. However, both botulism and E. coli, for instance, reside within our intestinal tracts as well as externally.

Indeed our health depends on a healthy balance between "friendly" and "unfriendly" microbes, with health practitioners both holistic and mainstream increasingly focusing on understanding the health of our internal biomes in relation to our overall health.

It is incredibly fascinating to think about this relationship between microbes, our health, and making cheese (and other cultured foods), and Sandor Katz, master fermenter, writes beautifully and extensively about the symbiotic and coevolutionary relationship between microbes and human existence in his book, *The Art of Fermentation*, a book I highly recommend. However, to return the focus to plant-based cheesemaking and food safety, I will leave you to explore this further on your own.

Particular strains of yeasts, moulds, and bacteria are encouraged to grow and are used to convert the medium (coconut, nut milk) into a cheese. As mentioned above, both friendly and unfriendly microbes are everywhere and within us, and in cheesemaking, the purpose of sanitization and maintaining a clean work area is to inhibit the unfriendly microbes and encourage the friendly, culturing microbes, the ones we want and need to do their work in making cheese.

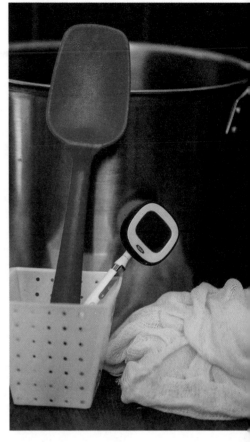

▲ Tools (1). CATHERINE DOWNES

While it is not possible, nor even necessarily desirable to eliminate all of them, it is absolutely essential in the cheesemaking process to ensure that your equipment, surfaces, forming molds, and so forth are clean and sanitized and that you have a safe, clean working and storage environment. Though it might seem obvious, here is a recommended approach for preparing your tools and surfaces.

Step 1: Washing

The first step is to make sure your tools, equipment, and surfaces are clean. This is the first step prior to sanitization. Use hot water and soap. Hot means not tepid, not lukewarm, but *hot*. Hot water and soap and a little elbow grease will remove any grime and unwanted debris from your utensils, the stove top, and working counter. Any household soap will work for this purpose.

Step 2: Rinse/Dry

After washing down your tools, equipment, and surfaces, it is important to wipe them down with a clean towel to remove any soapy residue. It is common to rinse your utensils after washing, so be sure to allow them to air dry fully. Air drying, if you are not using a dishwashing machine, is the best way to ensure that all moisture has evaporated. Moisture is the place where unwanted bacteria and microbes thrive and towel drying, rather than removing all moisture, actually can create a thin layer of pervasive moisture that can last for a long time, in addition to contributing unwanted fibres and potentially spreading microbes if you are not using a clean towel.

Step 3: Sanitizer

Only after the cleaning process can sanitization occur. I use a quaternary sanitizer or an acid sanitizer solution I purchase from Glengarry Cheese Company, Cultures for Health, or a local janitor's supply warehouse. Quaternary sanitizers are deemed food safe. I mix this at 30 milliliters to 1 liter of water. Using a bleach and water solution of 1 tablespoon (30 milliliters) to 3.8 litres of water, is also an effective sanitizer, though you should wait up to 45 minutes to allow chlorine to evaporate before placing any food element in contact with the sanitized surface. Chlorine will also destroy the helpful microbes that you want to work with.

After the washing process, use the sanitizing solution to wipe down utensils, forms, and surfaces on which you will handle any of the cheese-related ingredients. If using the bleach solution, allow the tools to rest and allow the chlorine to evaporate, or rinse in clean water and allow to air dry.

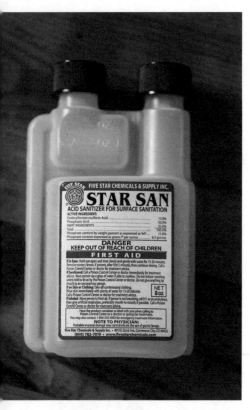

▲ Sanitizer. CATHERINE DOWNES

Although fermentation and culturing evolved from dubious circumstances and conditions, we can avoid some of the riskier elements of this incredibly beneficial practice by ensuring our work spaces are clean and ready to encourage healthy cultures.

Step 4: Hand Washing

Though your hands will be quite clean after cleaning and sanitizing your tools and surfaces, washing your hands before you begin directly working with ingredients is still important, and a good habit to develop.

Hand washing is often done hastily and without deep attention. However, as you are about to handle cultures and apply them to food ingredients, making sure your hands are as clean as possible is helpful.

Under warm running water rinse your hands, then add 3–5 milliliters of soap (if liquid). If using bar soap, make sure you lather it up quite well.

Rub your hands together well, making sure to wash your fingers, backs and palms of hands, and up to your wrists. Use a nail brush to scrub your nails, making sure to remove foreign debris. Take your time, sing a song to prolong the time you spend scrubbing your hands.

According to food safety guidelines from several nations, states and provinces, 15–30 seconds of vigorous handwashing under warm water with soap will be sufficiently effective.

After washing, be sure to rinse your hands well and dry them completely.

TOOLS AND EQUIPMENT

While each of the recipes will require a slightly different combination of equipment, there are some essential tools that you will need.

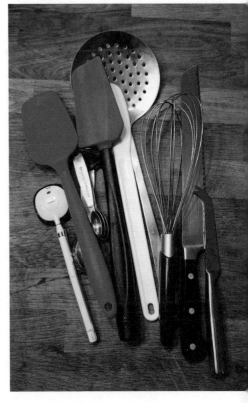

▲ Tools (2). CATHERINE DOWNES

Key Tools

- High-speed blender
- Wooden/silicone spoon and spatula
- Stainless steel stock pot, with thick cast bottom (use a medium sized pot, three to five liters, depending on size of batch you want to make)
- Glass or food-grade plastic bowl (medium sized, enough room to stir and mix if necessary)
- Probe thermometer
- pH meter
- Cheesecloth
- Nut milk bags
- Measuring cups
- Measuring spoons
- Mason jars, 500 ml to 1 L or for rejuvelac and kefir making
- Plastic or metal forms for shaping
- Wood boards
- Sushi mats/cheese mats
- Plastic wrap

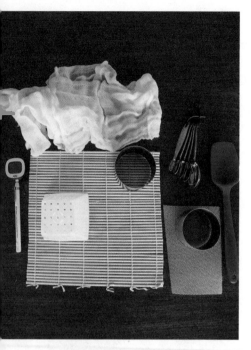

▲ Tools (3). CATHERINE DOWNES

Ingredients

Here are some of the essential ingredients you will use with the recipes and processes outlined in this book. As with the equipment above, you will not necessarily be using all of these ingredients in every recipe/process. This outline is to give you a broad idea of what you may want to keep on hand in your pantry should the urge strike you to make some cheese. Specific ingredients for particular cheese styles (i.e. figs, sundried tomatoes) will be mentioned in the individual recipe outlines.

- Wheat berries, for making rejuvelac* (farro, spelt, or quinoa may also be used)
- Coconut kefir (water kefir grains)*
- Probiotic capsules (read labels closely for source and vegan friendliness)*
- Sauerkraut brine*
- Miso*
- Traditional dairy cheese cultures: mesophilic direct set culture*
- Apple cider vinegar
- Lemon juice
- Vegetable rennet *
- Calcium chloride *

- Agar*
- Tapioca starch
- Nutritional yeast*
- Salt (non-iodized)
- Filtered water

- Cashews
- Almonds
- Sunflower seeds
- Walnuts
- Coconut milk

* See Appendix 1 for a list of ingredients and potential suppliers.

3

MAKING QUICK
NON-CULTURED CHEEZE

THIS CHAPTER PROVIDES a brief overview of some of the common approaches to creating do-it-yourself quick cheeze. Although some of these can be adapted and altered for a culturing approach, typically these types of cheeses are meant to be produced quickly, and to evoke a sense of cheese through the use of added ingredients to create familiar flavor and/or texture, rather than relying on the application of a culture and aging time to produce taste and texture.

Dairy cheese, for those who still choose to eat it, or for those who have sense memory from when they once did, has some particularly distinguishing characteristics. Texture, whether it be firm and smooth, soft and creamy, or somewhere between the two, is key. Aroma, which can be polarizing to some extent, in that some people do not like or appreciate the stronger funkier cheeses such as blue or limburger, is still a factor. Finally, taste. There is something about the combination of tangy, salty, and fatty that causes some people to virtually swoon when eating cheese and lament the prospect of giving it up.

Quick cheezes aim to capture some combination of these characteristics, often aiming at the most popular or most widely recognized realm of dairy-based cheese. Many plant-based cheeses now on the market attempt to simulate some of these. Tal Ronnen's Kite Hill,

Vtopia, Chao by Field Roast, Miyoko's Creamery (more artisanal than some of the others), Daiya, Earth Island, and Tofu Rella are some of the more broadly recognized names producing cultured or non-cultured plant-based cheeze. Cheddar slices, mozzarella, cream cheese, brie, and shredded cheese for nachos or pizza, are all available in one form or another.

Below I'll detail three base recipes that can be flavored as you wish. While these cheezes are not cultured, they can, with some care, be aged. I'll cover aging in detail at the end of recipes to which it applies. The three base recipes will provide you options for making soft, semi-soft and firm cheezes, which can be flavored as you prefer.

I am not providing a brie-style cheeze, as it is difficult to capture the internal creaminess of a dairy brie without culturing. The act of culture on the medium, consuming the sugars and altering the dairy protein structure, leads to the result, so I am avoiding that particular style here.

The following recipe for soft, semi-soft and firm cheese can be modified for personal preference. It is a dominant trend these days that people seek fast information and fast ways of doing things, and often, in my opinion, this leads to unsuccessful results especially with food. Making food, and cheese, is a way of reconnecting to process, to understanding through observation and patience. It is an opportunity to create some time for yourself, to slow things down a little, and to enjoy the act of doing something. Thus I've chosen to write these recipes in a manner that allows enough room for experimentation based around some key information with respect to the use of particular ingredients.

I have found this is a useful approach, if mildly provocative, as I find when people rely solely on recipes, they are not paying as close attention to the food and process itself. It is the marriage of recipe and user that yields the best results, and once you are using the culturing recipes, observation, patience and deeper involvement are necessary to good outcomes.

NON-CULTURED SOFT CHEEZE

This simple outline lists the basic steps required to make all of the below cheezes. You can use this as a simple quick reference guide, but I recommend that you closely review the recipes first.

1. Soak nuts
2. Drain nuts
3. Blend with clean, filtered water
4. Place in food grade bowl/container
5. Add seasoning/flavor (salt/acidity)
6. Drain in nut milk bag or through cheesecloth
7. Store in sealed container

SOFT CHEEZES

Although plant-based cheesemaking is still in its infancy and there is no formal nomenclature, soft cheezes are non-cultured and somewhere between spreads, dips, and pâtés in consistency.

Equipment required

- Jar or container for soaking cashews or sunflower seeds
- Sieve/colander for draining
- Measuring spoons
- High-speed blender
- Spatula
- Cheesecloth
- Container for storage

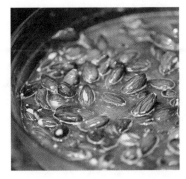

▲ Almonds soaking (soak all nuts or seeds you use). CATHERINE DOWNES

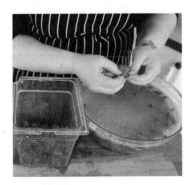

▲ Peeling almonds. CATHERINE DOWNES

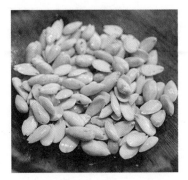

▲ Peeled almonds. CATHERINE DOWNES

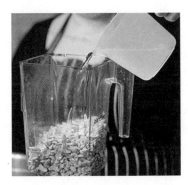

▲ Pouring filtered water into blender with nuts. CATHERINE DOWNES

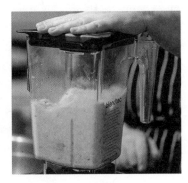

▲ Blending nuts. CATHERINE DOWNES

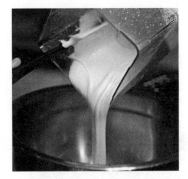

▲ Pouring blended nut mix into bowl. CATHERINE DOWNES

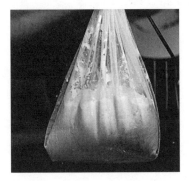

▲ Draining nut paste (blended, not cultured). CATHERINE DOWNES

WALNUT RICOTTA

This cheeze is not truly a ricotta, but does have a ricotta-type texture and is a great addition to pasta or zoodle dishes. It is a little outside of the core recipes I present here in that it is not as flexible in terms of multiple uses, but is a soft-style cheeze and meets raw food requirements.

Method

1. Soak the walnuts from 1 hour to overnight. Walnuts have quite a bit of tannin in their skins, giving them a slight bitterness. Soaking them longer helps to remove much of this bitter flavor.
2. Drain the walnuts and place the almond (or coconut) milk, lemon juice, salt, and nutritional yeast in the blender, add the walnuts, and start blending on low speed.
3. Increase the speed only moderately. You are not aiming to achieve a creamy texture, but rather a cottage cheese-style texture.
4. Scrape the mixture out of the pitcher and into a cheesecloth or nut milk bag and allow to drain for 1–2 hours.
5. Place the drained mixture in a sealed container. You can add garlic, parsley, or other herbs should you desire.
6. Keeps refrigerated for up to 5 days, walnuts will sour.

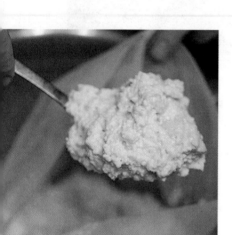

▲ Example of ricotta-style texture. CATHERINE DOWNES

▶ Finished almond ricotta in jars. Ricotta can be flavoured with herbs and fruit. COLIN MEDHURST

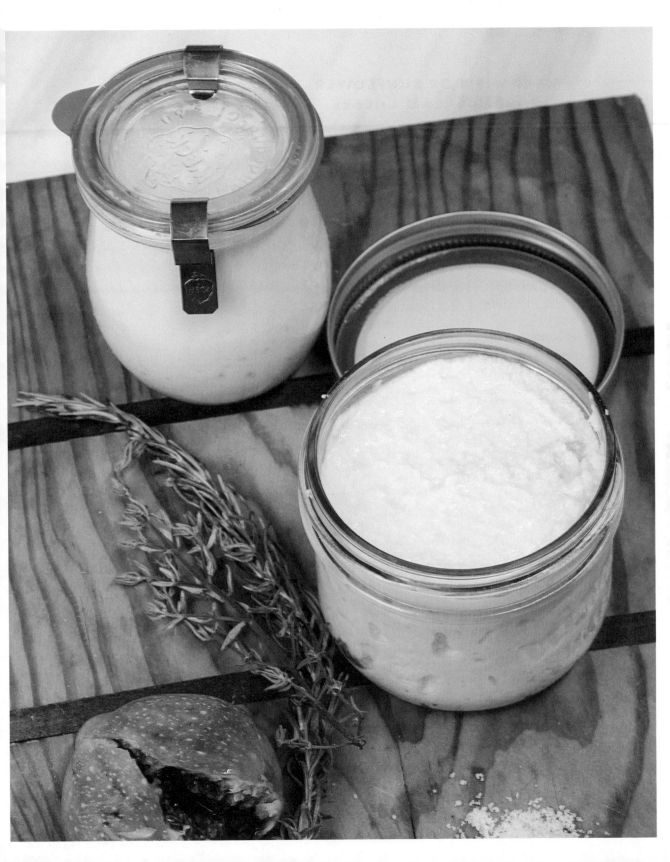

CASHEW OR SUNFLOWER SEED CREAM CHEEZE

INGREDIENTS

2 cups cashews or sunflower seeds (soaked)

2 tsp salt (use a good quality non-iodized salt, such as grey sea salt or pink Himalayan)

2–3 tbsp nutritional yeast (optional)

2 tbsp lemon juice (fresh squeezed is best, but not necessary)

2 tsp apple cider vinegar

Water to consistency

The consistency you seek is very smooth, creamy, and thick. This will take a bit of time, pulsing the blender, and scraping down the sides repeatedly, adding small amounts of water as you go, and gradually increasing speed. The amount of water you add will depend on how much moisture the nuts you are using contain, and how moist or soft you wish the cheeze to be. To achieve a firmer cheeze, add less water, and pulse and scrape more frequently.

Method

1. Soak the cashews or the sunflower seeds in a clean, sanitized container with filtered water and a tiny pinch of salt. Allow them to soak from 1 hour to overnight. However, if they soak overnight, they will be very soft, and the texture of the cheeze may be much more fluid than you desire.

   The primary reason for soaking nuts and seeds is not only to soften them but rather to remove some of the phytic acid which is the form in which nuts, seeds, legumes, and many plants store phosphorous. This is important for the plants born from these seeds and nuts, as it provides necessary energy for growth. Phytic acid assists in protecting seeds, legumes, and nuts from degradation until conditions are suitable for the sprouting and growing of the seed into its plant form. Along with phytic acid, there are a number of enzyme inhibitors in nuts and seeds. These prevent digestive and metabolic enzymes in humans and animals from being able to fully digest the nuts and seeds, thereby allowing many to pass right through (I think we've all seen seeds present in animal scat...).

   Soaking nuts and seeds in warm water with a little salt helps to deactivate the enzyme inhibitors and leach out some of the phytic acid thus allowing us to more easily digest them and obtain more of their nutritional value. The added bonus is that this makes blending nuts and seeds a whole lot easier.

2. After soaking, drain the nuts or seeds and rinse to remove any of the slimy residue which may be present. This is a result of the enzymes being leached and acting on the surface of the nuts or seeds.

3. If you have a food processor, place the nuts or seeds in the food processor and blend until as smooth as possible. There will still be some texture; don't worry too much about this, as you can refine it in the second blend. If you do not have a food processor, you will have to do a bit more work with your blender, pulsing, scraping, and adding small amounts of water to achieve smoothness.

4. After blending in the food processor, remove from the processor, using a spatula to get all of the paste out. Add all of the liquid components (i.e., lemon juice, vinegar) to a high-speed blender first, then the salt, nutritional yeast, and any of the flavoring elements that you wish to add. *Alternatively, if you wish to have some texture, you can reserve things such as figs, and add them at the end of the blending process or even turn them into the mixture by hand.*

5. Blend until smooth, adding small amounts of filtered water a little at a time. Take time to interrupt the blending process. Use a spatula to clear the sides and then add water. Be careful to not turn the blender on to highest speed immediately (an instinct many have). It is best to start at lower speeds to allow the blender blades to catch the material and then gradually turn the speed up, combining this with spatula scraping and small additions of water.

6. Blend until you reach the desired consistency. Also, as you blend, check the seasoning to see if you need to adjust any of the elements, particularly the salty and acidic ones. If needed, add more salt, vinegar, or lemon juice. Be careful to not add too much water at once, as you may possibly end up with more of a sauce than a cheeze, though this may not be a terrible outcome.

7. Once you have reached the texture you desire, scrape the mixture out of the blender and place inside a cheesecloth bag, (nut milk bags,

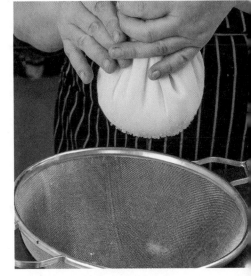

▲ Draining cheeze over bowl (1).
COLIN MEDHURST

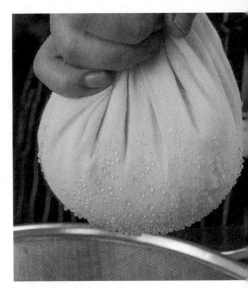

▲ Draining cheeze over bowl (2).
COLIN MEDHURST

or synthetic porous produce bags, are suitable alternatives). Hang the bag over a bowl and allow to drain for up to 4 hours at room temperature, or up to overnight in the refrigerator if you desire a firmer, drier cheeze.

8. After the cheeze has drained excess fluid, you can store in a container as is, covered and refrigerated, for up to 10 days. If you wish to dress it up for presentation at a party, or just for fun, you can place the cheeze mixture in a shaping mold, or hand shape the mixture, and then cover it in herbs, spices, mix herbs or dried fruit in, or whatever pleases you.

9. If you are aiming to make a firmer or drier cheeze, you will want to place the mixture in a cheesecloth lined ring mold or other shape molding device, place on a bamboo mat, and then on a wood board, and place in the refrigerator to allow excess moisture to evaporate.

Flavor options

1. Fig, tarragon and balsamic: add ⅓ cup chopped figs, dried, and 2 tbsp balsamic vinegar in place of the apple cider vinegar.

2. Roasted garlic, cracked pepper and rosemary: add ½ bulb of roasted garlic, ½ tbsp coarse cracked black pepper, and as much chopped fresh rosemary as you like.

3. Dill, mint, and lemon: add 4 tbsp chopped fresh dill, 2 tbsp chopped fresh mint, and zest of 1 lemon.

Again, this is a great base recipe to try with your own flavor combinations. Storage time for this cheeze is up to 10 days, properly covered or wrapped. With the absence of culture, the cashew may want to ferment on its own; don't be alarmed. If you find your batch getting a bit sharp tasting, it may be that the cashew paste has begun fermenting. So long as you have kept the container clean, not used your fingers to taste, or cross contaminated the mixture in some way, you can continue to use the cheeze if you like the evolving flavor profile.

If you avoid adding cooked ingredients to this core recipe it is suitable for raw food diet preferences.

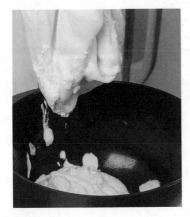

▲ Placing drained cheeze in bowl for mixing prior to mixing herbs. COLIN MEDHURST

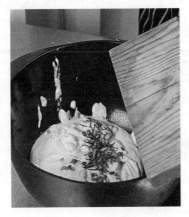

▲ Adding herbs to cheeze. But you can add dried fruit, or spices, or things such as sundried tomatoes or olives. COLIN MEDHURST

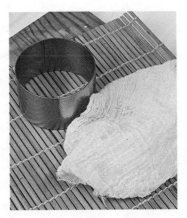

▲ Ring mold and cheesecloth for shaping cheese and cheeze. COLIN MEDHURST

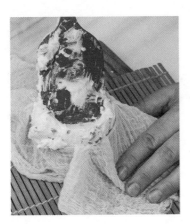

▲ Adding cheese or cheeze to cheesecloth-lined ring mold. COLIN MEDHURST

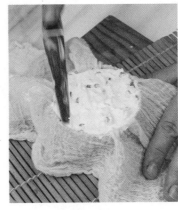

▲ Smoothing cheese or cheeze top. COLIN MEDHURST

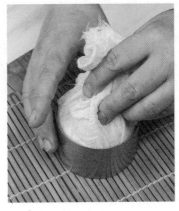

▲ Gathering and folding the cheese-cloth over the top of the cheese or cheeze. COLIN MEDHURST

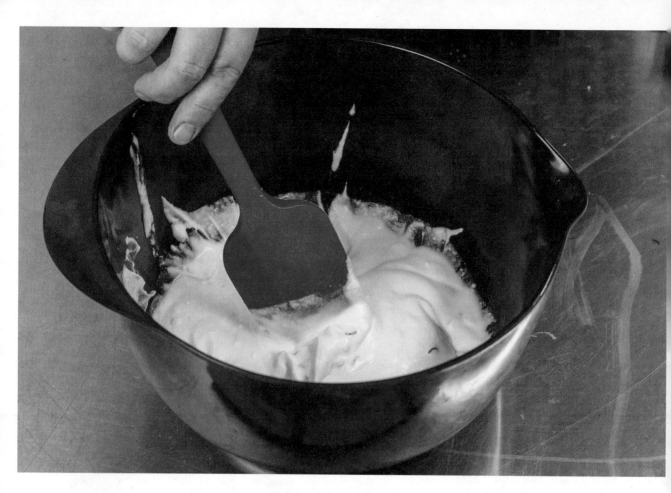

▲ Folding herbs into cheeze.

COLIN MEDHURST

▶ Pouring cheeze into cheesecloth.

COLIN MEDHURST

WAYS TO USE THIS CHEEZE

- sandwiches and toast
- in raw lasagne
- in baked vegan lasagne
- in ravioli

- scooped into small balls, and used in vegan caprese salads, or salads in general

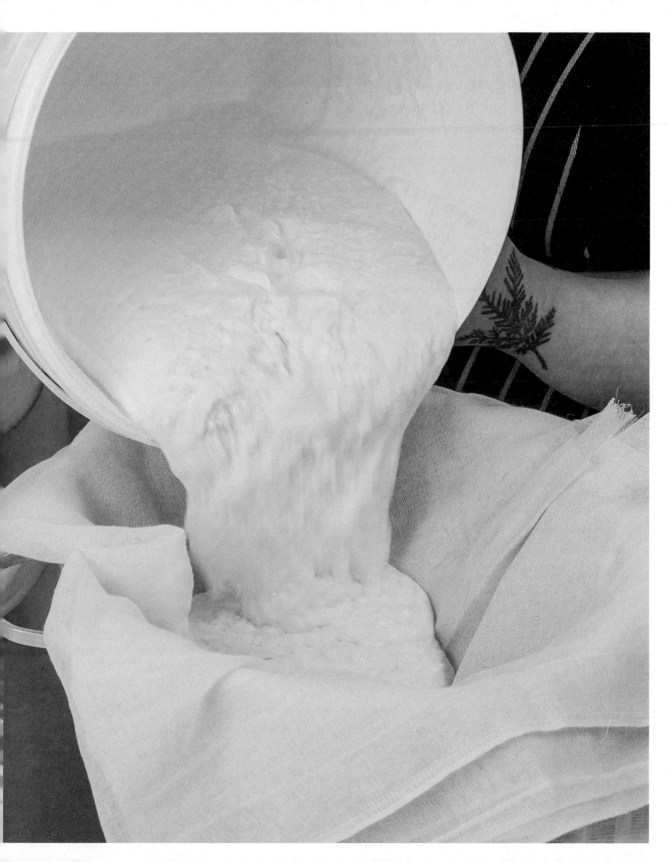

SEMI-SOFT CHEEZE
BASE RECIPE

EQUIPMENT

High-speed blender

Spatula

Wooden or silicone spoon

Thick cast sauce pot

Cheesecloth

Springform pan (or other circular mold) 6–8 inch (you can use other alternative forms, or loaf pans if you like)

INGREDIENTS

2 Cups cashews, soaked, OR 3 cups soaked and peeled almonds (you can also substitute macadamia nuts)

⅔ cup nutritional yeast

3 tsp salt

½ cup lemon juice or ⅓ cup apple cider vinegar

1 cup coconut milk (from can)

2 tbsp tapioca starch* (optional)

2 tsp powdered agar agar (powdered rather than flake)

1–1½ cups filtered water (for once the mixture goes into the pot)

Like the soft cheeze base, this is a base recipe which you can adapt to different flavors and densities. Semi-soft, for the purposes of my classification system, mirrors the texture style of some of the dairy-based cheeses that are also classified as semi-soft such as many of the blue cheeses, havarti, gouda, muenster, mozzarella, fontina, and Monterey jack.

Unlike all of the traditional cheeses, the cheeze base recipe below will not yield as many varieties as listed above, because of the lack of cultures, but it is very suitable for getting creative with flavors.

*Tapioca starch is optional, but if you are looking to create a cheeze that will have some stretchy texture under heat (i.e., melted), then tapioca starch does help. Since nuts and seeds do not have the same protein structure as dairy, it is a constant challenge to achieve the full-on meltability that occurs with dairy-based cheeses. Tapioca starch should not be replaced with potato, corn or arrowroot. Tapioca starch behaves very differently than the other starches, and does indeed impart stretchiness to mixtures.

Method

1. Soak cashews for 1 hour to overnight.

   If you are using almonds, use organic ones in skin. It is more work, but you will get better results. Soak the almonds in 6 cups of filtered water for a minimum of 3 hours to overnight. I use a little bit of very hot water to soak the almonds in as I find this helps in removing the skins. Keep in mind that almonds are less sweet than cashews so they will result in a different tasting cheese.

2. Place all ingredients, except the tapioca starch and the agar agar, into a high-speed blender starting with the liquids (coconut milk and lemon juice or vinegar). Start on low speed, then work your way up to

high speed. Stop periodically to scrape down the sides of the pitcher and continue repeating the blending and scraping process until very smooth. To judge smoothness, you can take a small amount of the mixture and rub it between your fingers. If you feel any graininess, continue the blending and scraping, and use a small amount of filtered water to assist with getting the texture smooth.

Most importantly, during this process be patient, as the blending process can take some time.

3. After you have finished the blending process, scrape all of the material from the blender pitcher into a thick cast pot. The texture will be quite thick, which means that when heating it will have a tendency to stick to the pot and be at risk of burning. Add the 1–1½ cups water to the pot, and stir in well with the wooden spoon.

4. Turn the element on to low heat and monitor the mixture closely. Taste-check for seasoning (namely salt, nutritional yeast and acidity). Stir frequently to prevent the nut paste from becoming burnt.

5. Add the agar and the tapioca starch (if you are using it), and stir thoroughly into the mixture to prevent lumps forming. Gradually increase the heat and stir frequently. Avoid the temptation to increase the heat rapidly and too high too soon. Tapioca starch likes to coagulate and will need time to bind with the rest of the mixture. Whisking will help the starch emulsify with the rest of the mixture.

6. As you are stirring and monitoring and gradually increasing the heat to medium-high, you should notice the texture becoming smooth and glossy. This will mean that the tapioca starch is well combined, and now you are paying attention to how the agar will respond. Agar needs to be heated at 186°F (85°C) for at least 5 minutes to "bloom," that is to become activated.

The reason this matters: agar is being used to set the cheeze mixture, as it cools, into a medium-firm substance. Agar is commonly used as a vegan alternative for gelatin in recipes; but, depending on how much and what kind (powdered or flake), will set more firmly than gelatine.

7. Continue stirring the mixture until it feels somewhat difficult, and you have surpassed the 5 minute blooming time for the agar. Taste test one more time, and adjust seasoning accordingly. The flavor is intended to be mild to moderate so that you can add other components if desired.

8. Turn the heat off and leave the mixture for a few minutes. Ready the springform pan by lining it with enough cheesecloth that the cloth spills over the edges and there is enough to fold over the top of the cheeze.

9. Pour the cheeze mixture into the springform pan and spread smooth with the spoon or offset spatula. Allow the mixture to cool to room temperature prior to setting in the refrigerator. The cheesecloth is important because it absorbs residual moisture from the mixture as it cools. Removing moisture will extend the shelf life of the cheeze.

10. After the cheeze has reached room temperature, pat it to test the firmness. It should be firm to touch, but have a very small amount of spring back. Keep in mind that as it continues to cool, it will firm up further.

   Store the cheeze in the refrigerator in the springform pan, and cover the top with cheesecloth. Do not cover it with plastic wrap or put it into a covered container, as this will lead to condensation developing and is a food safety risk as this moisture can become a prime environment for unwelcome microbes. Even though the cheeze has cooled to room temperature, it will take several more hours for all of the residual heat to evaporate.

   Allow this cheeze to fully cool and set overnight within the cheesecloth (you can use parchment or butter muslin to line the springform/mold). The next day check its firmness. Change the cheesecloth wrap (if you used cheesecloth; remove the parchment if you used parchment), remove the springform round, and store on a bamboo or wood board for 1–2 days more, as you allow a little moisture to continue evaporating. Make sure to flip or turn the cheeze every day, and to move to a dry board.

Modifications

Spicy hot pepper

Add ¼ cup very finely sliced hot peppers of choice, pickled or fresh. My preference is pickled: one, for flavor, and two, because they are less likely to impart foodborne pathogens. I also like to add 1 tsp powdered turmeric to change the colour of the cheeze. Add these ingredients when you add the cheeze mixture to the pot.

Smoked

While this particular cheeze mixture won't sustain an actual smoking process all that well (i.e., being smoked over wood chips), you can impart a smoky element in a number of ways.

Add 1 tbsp smoked salt in place of the salt in the recipe, 2 tsp smoked paprika, and 1 tsp liquid smoke.

These elements should be added during the blending process. You can, and should, adjust them to your preference. If you want it quite smoky you should also add more nutritional yeast and increase the acidity slightly by adding either pasteurized (bottled) lemon juice or vinegar.

It ultimately comes down to your taste preference so be sure to taste frequently during the process, and gradually adjust the key elements of salt, umami (nutritional yeast), and acidity (lemon juice or apple cider vinegar) as you work.

Apricot or cranberry

Add ½ cup chopped dried apricot or dried cranberry, and ⅛ cup lemon zest. Optional: add ½ cup white wine such as a Riesling or Viognier. Add these elements when you add the cheeze mixture to the pot.

For all three amendments, be sure to follow the rest of the process as outlined in the base recipe.

For an additional presentation element, while the cheeses are cooling add dried fruit or slices of hot pepper into the surface.

> **WAYS TO USE THIS CHEEZE**
> - sandwiches, pizza, flatbread, (raw or cooked)
> - torn into chunks in salads
> - melted on baked potatoes
> - any way you like

FIRM/HARD CHEEZE BASE

EQUIPMENT/TOOLS REQUIRED

High-speed blender
Spatula
Wooden or silicone spoon
Thick cast sauce pot
Springform pan or other
    form (i.e., loaf pan)
Thermometer
Cheesecloth

INGREDIENTS

2 cups cashews, or 3 cups
    almonds, or 2 cups
    macadamia nuts
2½ tsp salt
⅓ cups apple cider vinegar
2 tbsp miso*
¼ cup nutritional yeast
1 cup coconut milk
1½ cup water
3 tbsp tapioca starch
    (optional)
1½ tbsp agar agar
    (powdered, not flake)

This base is designed to allow you to create a quite firm cheeze and as with the other cheeze bases, it enables you to create a cheeze that suits your preference and style.

*Note that though miso is a fermented food that can be used to assist in creating cultured cheeses, it is used in this recipe to add umami, or depth of flavor, to the cheese base.

Method

1. Soak the cashews, almonds, or macadamia nuts in filtered water, for a minimum of 1 hour.

2. If using almonds, peel them. Skins can be composted.

3. Add all ingredients except the water, tapioca starch, and agar to a high-speed blender. Remember to add the liquids first.

4. Beginning on low speed, gradually increase speed, making sure to stop periodically and scrape the mixture down the sides of the pitcher. Repeat this process as often as necessary to achieve a smooth, creamy texture. If necessary, use small amounts of filtered water to aid in achieving the desired consistency.

5. Once you have achieved a very creamy, non-grainy texture, pour the mixture into a thick cast sauce pot, making sure to use a spatula to scrape out as much of the mixture as possible. Add the water, and begin on low heat.

6. Stirring frequently to ensure that the water is well combined with the mixture, gradually increase the heat. Add the tapioca starch. In order to prevent clumping of the tapioca starch, stir continuously. Mix the agar with about ⅓ cup water, then pour into the mixture. Stir to combine.

7. Do not allow the mixture to boil, and while stirring watch for the texture to begin to get shiny and smooth.

8. Remember, agar needs to be exposed to a temperature of at least 186°F (86°C) for five minutes to bloom; use a thermometer to check the temperature. Stirring will prevent the agar from clumping, and ensure that it is spread through the mixture evenly.

9. Once the mixture is very thick and difficult to stir remove from the heat and pour into a cheesecloth-lined small mold of your choice (springform, loaf pan, etc).

10. Allow it to cool to room temperature. Fold the top of the cheesecloth over the cheeze and set in the refrigerator. After 12 hours, or the next day, remove from the form, change the cheesecloth and let it rest on a wood or bamboo board to dry. Flip the cheeze after 6 hours or so, and repeat this process over a couple of days. Moisture will continue to evaporate, and the more that evaporates, the firmer the cheeze will become and the longer its shelf life.

11. Keep the cheeze wrapped in cheesecloth for at least 3 days (change it once a day if particularly damp). Once surface is dry to touch, not damp, wrap tightly in plastic wrap. Now that the cheeze is fully cooled, and most of the inherent moisture has evaporated, the plastic wrap will prevent continued evaporation (slow dehydration … we've all seen the shrivelled piece of vegetable or rock-hard dairy cheese in the bottom of a refrigerator drawer) as well as potential cross-contamination from other items stored in the fridge.

12. However, if you would like the cheeze to end up firmer, you can continue to air-dry on a bamboo mat, in the refrigerator. Make sure to flip the cheeze every day, and to change the bamboo mat every 2 days. Ensure that you can do this in the fridge safely, without risk of cross-contamination from items such as meat, poultry, fish or dairy. If this is a risk, avoid further air-drying the cheeze.

13. The cheeze is good for up to 2 weeks, properly stored in the refrigerator.

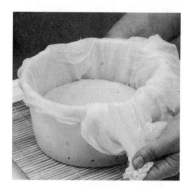

▲ Cheeze in cheesecloth inside mold. COLIN MEDHURST

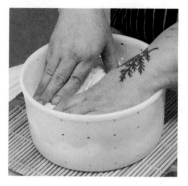

▲ Folding cheesecloth over top of the cheeze. COLIN MEDHURST

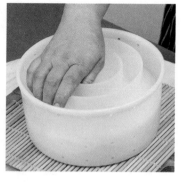

▲ Placing a "follow" on top of the cheeze. This allows weight to be placed on top to allow for pressing of the cheeze, and removal of moisture. COLIN MEDHURST

Modifications

This base is a great one for experimenting with adding other elements such as herbs, spices, and dried fruit.

Smoky cheddary cheeze

Add 2 tsp turmeric, 2 tsp smoked paprika, 2 tsp smoked salt, 1 tsp liquid smoke (optional depending on smoky preference), 1 tbsp extra nutritional yeast, 1 tbsp extra apple cider vinegar.

Add all of the elements at the blending stage. Taste after adding each ingredient to ensure that the mixture meets your flavor preference.

Roasted garlic peppercorn

Add ½ bulb of roasted garlic, peeled and roughly chopped and 1 tbsp coarse black peppercorn and 2 tsp pink peppercorn.

Apricot

Add ⅓ cup chopped dried apricot, 1 tbsp extra nutritional yeast, ¼ cup dry white wine. Reduce the amount of apple cider vinegar in base recipe by half. Add the nutritional yeast and white wine during the blending process. Fold the chopped apricot into the mixture after it has been heated.

Note Dried fruit have sugars, and sugars naturally want to ferment. Be sure to add the fruit at the lowest temperature possible. The fruit will also shorten the shelf life of the cheeze, but that is okay, you will probably eat it all before two weeks anyway!

Pseudo-blue

Blue cheeses are pungent, tangy, salty. Though this will not achieve the funkiness of a true blue as it is not even cultured, it is a fun cheeze just for appearances and the added nutritional benefit of blue-green algae.

After you have made the base, and are about to pour it into a form, add 1 tbsp blue-green algae (I use E3Live) a little at a time, swirling it into the mix, but do not overstir or you will end up with the entire cheeze looking bluish, rather than giving the impression of veins.

Sassy and spicy

Add ⅛ cup very finely sliced hot peppers, 2 tsp chipotle, 1 tsp smoked paprika, and 1 tsp sriracha or other hot sauce. Add all of these, except the sliced hot peppers, during the blending process. This one depends entirely on how spicy you like things. I like very spicy so I tend to veer toward the hotter end of the spectrum. Roasted garlic also works well with this as well as a sprinkling of black sesame seeds.

NOTES ON INGREDIENTS

Tapioca Starch

Tapioca starch, as mentioned earlier, cannot be replaced in these recipes by other starches. Starches, while sharing in common the

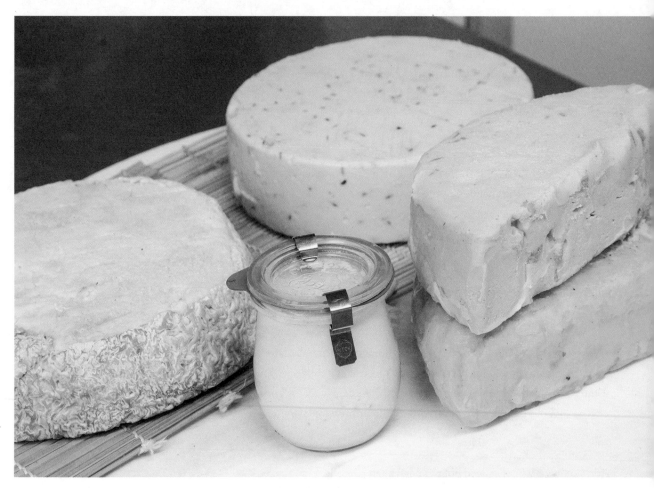

▲ Variety of finished or drying cheezes and cheese. COLIN MEDHURST

fact that they are carbohydrates, do not all perform the same tasks equally. Arrowroot and potato starch are reliable thickening agents but do not provide any pull or stretchiness when heated. Since the purpose of adding a starch to this cheeze base is to allow it to melt in a similar fashion to traditional cheeses, it is therefore important to use the starch listed in the base recipe, tapioca.

Tapioca starch is used because when heated it provides stretchiness, one of the main elements of plant-based cheeze/cheese that is very difficult to replicate because the protein structure and protein/carbohydrate matrix of nut and seed bases is very different from dairy.

In these recipes I try to keep the use of tapioca starch to a minimum, and leave it as optional. I do not tend to use it myself very often, as I prefer to avoid using a lot of fillers and am not necessarily trying to copy traditional cheeses, but this is my personal preference. However, just to put it into perspective, if you have ever had bubble tea, you have consumed tapioca, as the bubbles in the tea are made of it.

Adding Tapioca Starch to Recipes

There are a few ways to add tapioca starch to recipes. Here are some suggested ways to work with tapioca.

- Add the measured amount of tapioca directly to the recipe mixture. In the case of cheeze recipes in which it is optional, do this just after the mixture starts to heat up. The mixture will become more fluid and therefore absorb the tapioca more readily with less clumping. Consistent stirring is essential to this method.
- Add the measured amount of tapioca to the mixture at blending time. This will ensure full inclusion, but will not eliminate the need to stir consistently. As you heat the mixture up, with the starch already included, it will want to thicken very quickly and will become clumpy.
- Make a slurry. A slurry is a mixture of starch and water, and is a very helpful way of including starches to soups, stews, and other cooked or heated recipes which you want to thicken. Use ⅓ cup water, preferably warm-hot, to 1 Tbsp starch and whisk together well before adding to the gently warming mixture. As you pour the slurry into the mixture, stir frequently.

Working with Agar Agar

Agar agar (or as referred to here, just agar) is derived from algae, and is the combination of polysaccharide and pectin molecules. It is a structural component of cell walls in algae and is released upon cooking. Agar is used in numerous applications, including in vegan and vegetarian cooking instead of gelatine.

There are two common forms of agar available commercially, powder and flakes. I recommend using the powdered form in these recipes as it is easier to use, requires less cooking time, and provides a nice firm set.

Adding Agar

Understanding agar

If you have not used agar before, I recommend playing with it first, just to get comfortable with the material. Place 1 cup of water in a sauce pan, add 2–4 teaspoons of agar, and bring to a boil. Agar, as mentioned earlier, requires exposure to heat (up to 186°F [86°C]) for a minimum of 5 minutes, before it will "bloom," or become activated.

You will need to stir or whisk it as it comes to a boil, and this is a great opportunity to observe it change as it is heated. The fluid will become slightly opaque and more gelatinous. Once this happens you know it will set when removed from heat.

A useful trick from jelly and jam making is the "cold plate test." Put a plate in the freezer or refrigerator and allow it to become quite cold. After you have heated the agar and maintained it at the right temperature for the right amount of time, take a spoonful and drop it onto the cold plate. It should cling to the plate almost immediately rather than running like a loose fluid.

This tells you that as it cools it will become firm or set.

Adding agar to cheeze recipes

Directly: You can add the powdered agar directly to the recipe mixture once it is in the pot. As with adding tapioca starch, you will need to stir frequently and monitor the temperature. Use a thermometer and do not raise the heat too quickly.

As mixture: Add the measured amount of agar to ½–⅔ cup water. Bring the mixture to a boil while stirring, and allow it to cook for 5 minutes at a sustained temperature of 186°F (86°C). Pour the mixture into the heated cheeze mixture and stir frequently. Continue heating the cheeze mixture and stirring for several minutes

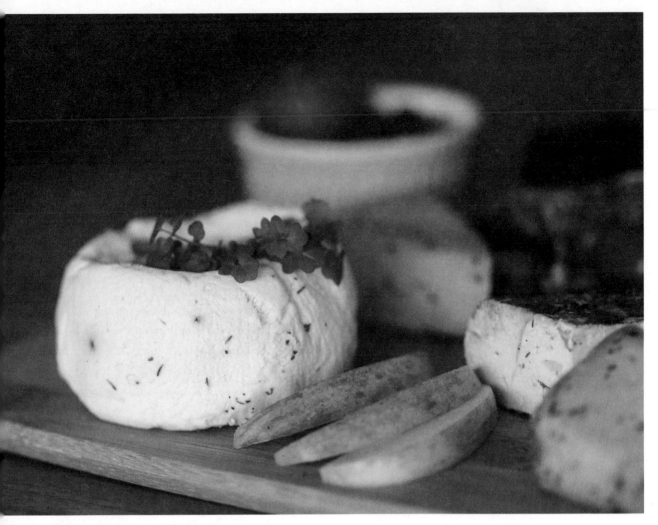

▲ Blue Heron cocochevre. CATHERINE DOWNES

to ensure that the agar mixture is fully integrated into the recipe. Alternatively, you can add the cheeze mixture to the agar and whisk it in. Testing which method works best for you will determine which approach you prefer.

If it clumps or feels too thick, you can always add small amounts of filtered water to loosen the mixture. On occasion, I have also blended the mixture after heating to achieve a completely smooth texture.

4

MAKING AND USING PLANT-BASED CULTURES

FERMENTATION AND CULTURING are related processes; they both rely on the activity of friendly microbes in altering a single food item or combination of food items from one state (raw) to another. We enjoy the results of fermentation in a number of products: beer, wine, sourdough bread, sauerkraut, kimchi, tempeh, kombucha, and sour pickles are just some of the most obvious ones. Fermentation of these products primarily refers to lactofermentation. This means that the fermentation activity is primarily the result of lactic acid-producing bacteria such as lactobacillus. These bacteria acidify the food, both preserving it and making it rich in probiotics.

Many of the things we ferment this way rely on naturally occurring bacteria and are thus a form of "wild" fermentation. For a more comprehensive discussion on the topic of wild fermentation, Sandor Katz's *Wild Fermentation* and *The Art of Fermentation* are outstanding references. Certainly there can be an element of wild fermentation in plant-based cheesemaking, but I will highlight that in the relevant recipes.

Culturing also relies on the use of bacteria, often many of the same ones as in fermentation, but it also uses yeasts, molds, and other bacteria. The formal distinction between fermentation and culturing may be flexible, but for the purposes of cheesemaking it is significant, in that culturing also implies active involvement from an outside source, in this case the cheesemaker. The cheesemaker controls the amount of time the medium is exposed to cultures, the temperature and humidity at which the cheese ages and ripens, and how to slow or alter the aging process. All of these things rely on understanding how the cultures (bacteria, yeasts, molds) like to function best.

In both traditional cheesemaking and the processes I employ, acidification of the medium is achieved through applying a lactic acid bacterial culture. Therefore, you will need a few basic plant-based culturing mediums. These culturing mediums are the by-products of fermenting processes on particular ingredients, such as wheat berries in the production of rejuvelac.

Acidification of the medium is crucial in culturing and fermentation. This action of culture on medium gives yogurt, kefir, and cheeses that tangy, sour taste. This first step of acidification commonly involves lactobacillus (a bacteria named for its willingness to feed on dairy sugars), but will also involve other lacto strains and friendly microbes. Lactobacilli reside on the surfaces of most things grown in the ground, and are responsible for the sour taste of sauerkraut (fermented cabbage), kimchi, and sour pickles.

Lactobacilli also reside within our digestive systems, and without them we would have an incredibly difficult time digesting many foods. The cultures used to create fermented foods have longstanding evolutionary relationships with the human digestive system, and are also the subject of interest when nutritionists, dieticians, and naturopaths refer to pro- and prebiotic activity, and healthy gut flora.

Without the application of the starter culture, the medium will not be acidified and will be prone to contamination by the growth of unwelcome microbes. In some cheeses, both dairy- and plant-based, only a single culture is used in the process, while others may involve using other cultures at different stages, such as washing a rind with a culture to create a surface-ripened cheese, or adding a culture to the medium at a later stage to stop the action of the first culture and allow a different flavor or texture to evolve. As this is an introductory book regarding the use of cultures, I will not delve too deeply into all of the ways in which cultures can be used.

Since cultures are living organisms they must be grown and used with care, a reminder that sanitizing your equipment and tools is critical and cannot be overemphasized. Make sure that all containers you will use in making rejuvelac or kefir are washed, sanitized, and air dried thoroughly.

REJUVELAC

Rejuvelac is the fermented fluid produced by the soaking and then fermentation of grains such as wheat berries (soft), buckwheat groats, quinoa, rye, farro, spelt, millet, and even rice. As a lactic acid-rich fluid, rejuvelac is often consumed by health-conscious vegans and vegetarians as a way of maintaining healthy digestive systems. As a tool in cheesemaking, rejuvelac provides a lactic acid-rich starter culture which can be used to acidulate (make acidic) a nut- or seed-based mylk/paste. This is significant, as the use of a lactic acid or starter culture is an essential component of the definition of cheese. A big difference between using a lactic acid starter culture such as rejuvelac versus the kind used in traditional cheesemaking is that those are usually dried and used in powdered form.

Each grain produces a culture which will have differing levels of culturing potency, strength of smell, and flavor. Wheat berries make a particularly strong rejuvelac, which is highly effective for culturing some nut pastes, but I have found it useful to explore using other types of rejuvelac in specific combinations. For instance when culturing almond paste, I have found it preferable to use a farro rejuvelac, as the stronger wheat berry one, in combination with the sulfur compounds of almonds, can yield a particularly strong odor, and a tendency to overculture, creating an almost unpleasant flavor.

MAKING REJUVELAC

In order to make rejuvelac several steps need to be followed closely. The following steps for wheat berry rejuvelac can be used with the other rejuvelac choices.

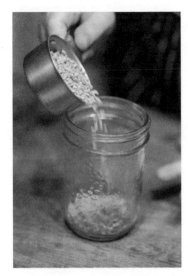

▲ Wheat berries in glass jar for sprouting. CATHERINE DOWNES

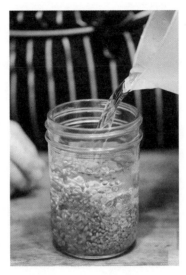

▲ Adding water to wheat berries. CATHERINE DOWNES

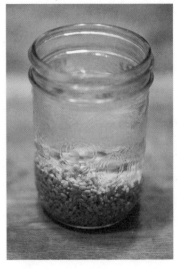

▲ Water-covered wheat berries. CATHERINE DOWNES

Step 1: Purchasing Your Wheat Berries

Ensure that your wheat berries are organic, soft, not the hard variety and most importantly, not irradiated. Irradiation of grains, legumes, nuts, and seeds is common, ostensibly to prolong shelf-life. However, the result also inhibits the sprouting ability of nuts, seeds, grains, and legumes, preventing the release of the necessary enzymes, because the lactobacilli which would normally be present have been destroyed.

As you practice making rejuvelac and trying different grains to make it, you may want to make a few different batches each using a different grain and set up a comparison test, to see which grain produces your favorite rejuvelac, as determined by taste, odor and activity.

Step 2: Sprouting

Place the washed, organic wheat berries in a sanitized 1 liter jar, and fill with filtered water to ⅔ full. *Filtered water is important as the chlorine that is in many urban water systems may inhibit the sprouting of the seeds.*

Chlorine will evaporate after 45 minutes, so if you do not have a filter, you can measure out your water and allow it to sit out while you wash the seeds and sanitize the jar.

Cover the jar with a sprouting mesh or cheesecloth, held in place with an elastic band.

Allow the wheat berries to soak for 24 hours at room temperature. After 24 hours, drain off the water, leaving the berries in the jar. Rinse and refill the jar, and repeat this process 2–3 more times a day, until the berries begin to sprout.

The importance of rinsing and draining off the water during the first 2–3 days of the sprouting process cannot be overstated. Rinsing and draining off the initial sprouting water eliminates phytic acid. A common concern about the use of rejuvelac as a commercial culturing agent is the troublesome bacteria, listeria, which has been found present in standing water, hence reinforcing the need to monitor the sprouting process closely.

Step 3: Fermentation

After the wheat berries have begun to sprout and have visible tails showing, strain off the water and place the sprouted berries in a jar large enough to allow air to circulate. Using a 4:1 ratio of water to sprouted berries, fill the jar with filtered water and cover with fresh cheesecloth, held in place by a tight rubber band or otherwise secured.

Allow the sprouted wheat berries to ferment at room temperature for 2–3 days. Monitor the progress. You will be looking for the fluid to become slightly cloudy, and for little bubbles to begin forming. The formation of bubbles indicates the bacteria are active and that the fluid is becoming rich in probiotics.

Rejuvelac should smell and taste slightly citrusy, though this will depend on the grain you use. Don't be surprised if you make a batch and it has a stronger, lightly cheesy-like odor, depending on the grain. The stronger smelling rejuvelacs tend to come from the wheat berry, spelt and farro grains. Strain the fluid off into another clean, sanitized jar and keep it covered in the refrigerator. The fluid can be kept for at least one week, but check it regularly to ensure that it still has the right odour and flavor. If you notice a lack of bubbles or that it starts to develop a funky, somewhat unpleasant odor, discard it.

The sprouted grain can be reserved to start a second batch of rejuvelac, which will take less time to make than the first batch. It is possible to reuse the sprouted grain one more time after this; however, it is likely that subsequent batches of rejuvelac will be less pleasant smelling and tasting, and less probiotically robust. The sprouted grain can also be eaten and, of course, used in compost.

While many people make rejuvelac for the purpose of consuming it as a beverage (I do as well), my preference is using it as a starter culture in making some plant-based cheeses and yogurts. Some of the easy, one to two day-cultured chevre- and ricotta-style cheeses I make use a rejuvelac culture, and those processes will be detailed later.

An important consideration for the use of rejuvelac is that it can be used in raw food applications without undermining the raw food guidelines. The limitations of rejuvelac are that it tends to impart a single level of flavor, and is not suitable for long-duration culturing.

KEFIR: COCONUT, CASHEW, ALMOND

Kefir (fed on cashew or coconut) is another plant-based culture that I use frequently, including as a single culture, or as the second acidification culture for some cheeses.

A fermented beverage, traditionally understood to be made from cultured dairy (cow, sheep, goat), kefir originates from Eastern Europe. It is tangy, fizzy, and naturally carbonated via the culturing process, with the consistency of a thin yogurt. This probiotic

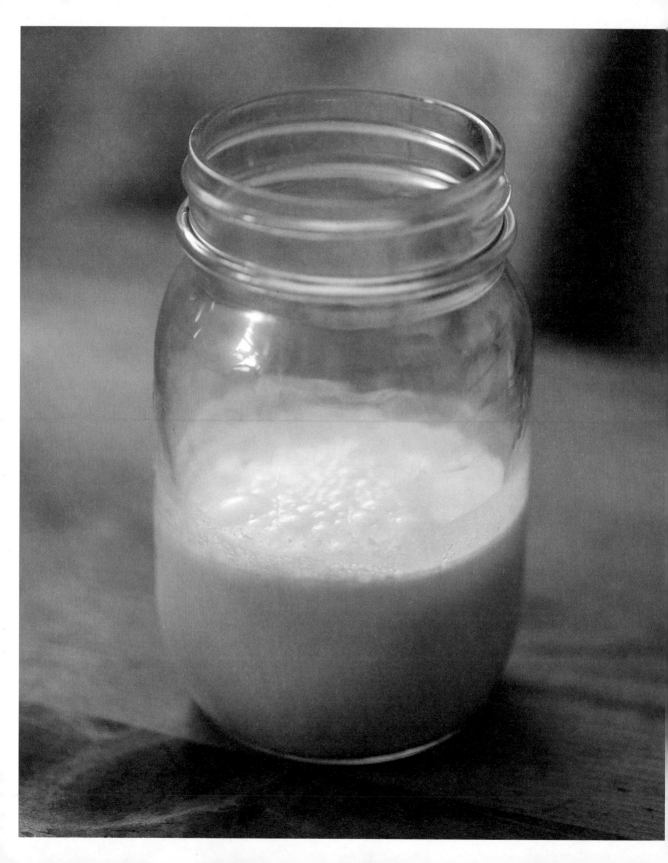

beverage is well understood to have significant positive health impacts on the digestive system. While dairy kefir is now fairly broadly available, currently there is no commercially available plant-based kefir, with the exception of water kefir, which is found primarily in health-focused specialty shops and restaurants.

The exception is Cultures for Health, an online store and education source for fermenting and culturing aficionados, based in the United States, is now selling kefir and yogurt cultures trained on non-dairy medium.

As I'm allergic to dairy, in addition to having chosen to live a plant-based lifestyle, I wanted to make a plant-based version of kefir and I began experimenting with this process over two years ago.

My first experiment was in converting some dairy-fed kefir grains given to me by a friend. Kefir grains are somewhat gelatinous looking in appearance, almost clear. They are composed of bacteria and yeasts, just as kombucha mother and vinegar mothers are, though the strains of bacteria and yeasts may vary. In order to identify which kefir feed I would want to work with most I set up to test several kefir options: cashew, almond, coconut, coconut water, and water.

With the assistance of Katie, a stage in the Graze kitchen, we set out to see if we could (1) successfully train the dairy-fed kefir grains onto a plant-based medium, and (2) make a kefir/yogurt/probiotic beverage that would work successfully as a starter for further cheese tests.

Dividing the grain into 5 different 1 liter jars, we added 2 cups of each test medium to each of the 5 jars (1 jar coconut milk, 1 jar cashew milk, etc.). We also added 1 tbsp of maple syrup, to help feed the kefir grains. We then kept the jars with lids in a container and set it on top of the convection oven where it was warm but not hot (maintaining 100°F [38°C]), and left them to culture for 24 hours.

After 24 hours, the coconut milk had very quickly cultured, with the kefir grain having multiplied quickly. We were able to strain

◀ Coconut kefir. CATHERINE DOWNES

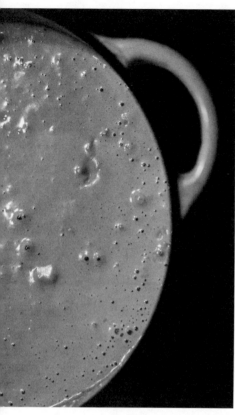

▲ Culturing coconut milk with kefir grain. CATHERINE DOWNES

off the coconut milk and save the grain for making another jar of coconut milk kefir in which we used less maple syrup. We repeated the coconut milk process two more times until the kefir grain was trained onto just coconut milk, with no added sweetener.

With each subsequent batch we saved the grain and evaluated the results of the cultured coconut milk for texture, taste, and that bright, somewhat effervescent quality of kefir beverages. Also, because the goal was to produce kefir grain fed only plant-based mediums, we discarded the first two rounds of the kefir. After batches three and four we reserved grain by straining the coconut milk through very fine mesh sieves in order to retrieve some of the grain.

We added the reserved grain to a small amount of coconut milk with a small amount of maple syrup, in order to store the kefir culture for a longer period of time in the refrigerator.

Frequent culturing will still result in a kefir product, but the grain will become very small and integrated into the beverage.

Now, for the other kefir efforts. The cashew and almond milks we made ourselves, in order to avoid the extra stabilizers and to be able to control the amount and kind of sweetener that we wanted to use. The cashew milk was a success, but did take a little longer (36 hours) to culture to the same degree of tanginess or sharpness as the coconut milk. It produced a thicker substance than the coconut milk, more like a very soft yogurt. The kefir grain, however, was much smaller, and we were not able to culture subsequent batches of cashew kefir as quickly as the coconut milk.

For the purposes of being able to maintain a supply of cashew kefir, we decided to culture cashew milk using coconut milk kefir as a starter. This worked well, and is still the method I use when making larger batches of cheeses.

The almond milk was more challenging. Of the milks, it took the longest, and had the least pleasant taste. This could be a result of the culture struggling with the sulfur compounds in almonds. We found that adding 2 tbsp maple syrup to 1 liter almond milk gave the kefir grain more to feed on, and resulted in a better tasting product.

As with the cashew kefir, if I am making large batches of cheese that require almond kefir starter, I start my almond milk kefir with starter from one of my coconut milk kefir batches. The coconut milk kefir is a highly consistent performer and requires little prodding to become acidic; therefore it works well for acidifying other mediums. It also has the longest shelf life — more than 30 days, refrigerated in a glass jar, and fed a little coconut sugar or maple syrup approximately once a week.

Lastly, with respect to the coconut water and water kefir tests, these took longer than all of the milks. The weaning process started with higher amounts of maple syrup (our sweetener of choice, though some people use raw cane sugar), with less and less in subsequent batches until we found the minimum we could use and still get the results we were seeking. I will often use water kefir as a starter in cheeses if I am concerned about allergies to coconut.

Since the coconut milk kefir is one I find quite easy to produce and replicate, and use frequently, I am including two processes for making it.

Note If you have not done a lot of culturing in your home such as making kefir, kombucha or sauerkraut, then don't be disappointed if the first couple of efforts don't go quite as well as you would like. Culturing compounds that use a starter grain, such as vinegar, kombucha, and even kefir, are aided by the presence in the air of naturally occurring bacteria such as acetobacter.

Frequent culturing activity will build up the presence of different types of bacteria and yeasts present in your home culturing environment. Think of it as your personal home micro-ecology.

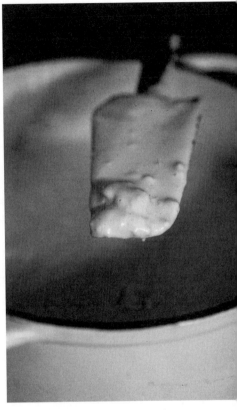

▲ Kefir grain lifted out of culture.
CATHERINE DOWNES

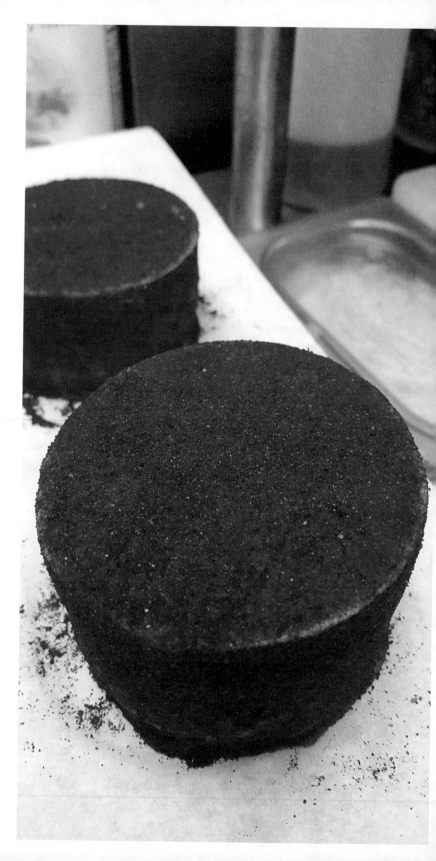

► Kefir cultured Blue Heron Creamery paprika rinded cheddar. AUTHOR

Method

1. Place the coconut milk in the refrigerator for a couple of hours to encourage the separation of the water from the fat. I do this because in cheesemaking I am not looking to make a drinkable beverage; I am seeking thickness and creaminess. If you just want to make a drinkable beverage, then there is no need to separate the water and fat.

2. Pre-heat oven to 100°F (38°C). Turn the heat off and leave the oven light on. This will provide enough ambient heat to maintain the right temperature for culturing.

3. Remove the coconut milk from the cans and place into a clean, sanitized bowl. Pour the fluid into a storage container, and save to use in cooking.

4. Place the kefir starter of choice and the maple syrup in the coconut milk and stir gently. Fill a clean, sterilized jar with the mixture, cover with a lid, and place the jar inside the oven. Allow to culture for 12–36 hours. Check after 12 hours.

> **INGREDIENTS**
> 500 ml of full-fat coconut milk (for cheese-making I only use full-fat coconut milk)
> 1 tbsp maple syrup, organic
> ½ pkg of coconut kefir culture (which can purchased from Cultures for Health) **or**
> ½ pkg water kefir grains **or**
> 2 tbsp of water kefir with grains **or**
> 2 tbsp kefir from a dairy source (if you are not concerned about using this as a starter).

You should observe small bubbles of activity within the coconut milk. Using a clean spoon, taste the kefir. It should taste slightly sour, which is what you want.

I culture my kefir closer to 36 hours, as I am using it primarily as a culturing agent in my cheese processes, and I'm seeking a high proportion of probiotic activity and sharpness for culturing other mediums.

The strength of the culture you want is up to you. But if you are culturing for longer periods of time, it is critical to make sure that the culturing temperature of 100–105°F (38–40°C) is maintained throughout the process. Using a yogurt maker is an excellent way to maintain consistent heat.

HEATING THE COCONUT MILK IN ADVANCE

INGREDIENTS

500 ml full-fat coconut milk (for cheesemaking I only use full-fat coconut milk)

1 tbsp maple syrup, organic

½ pkg of coconut kefir culture (which can be purchased from Cultures for Health) or

½ pkg water kefir grains **or**

2 tbsp water kefir with grains **or**

2 tbsp kefir from a dairy source (if you are not concerned about using this as a starter).

This process involves heating the coconut milk to just below the boiling point and then holding it at this heat point for up to 15 minutes. This allows some of the water to evaporate without scalding or cooking the coconut milk. I've also found that this results in a much thicker kefir or yogurt when finished culturing.

Method

1. In a heavy cast sauce pot, add the 500 ml full-fat coconut milk.
2. Bring the coconut milk up to 180°F (82°C); you must use a thermometer to test.
3. Do not allow the coconut milk to boil.
4. Remove from heat.
5. Transfer the coconut milk into a metal bowl or leave in the pot.
6. Place the pot or bowl over ice and stir frequently, at least every 15 minutes, to ensure that the hot coconut milk at the bottom comes to the top and the mixture can cool evenly.
7. Check the temperature every 30 minutes. When the coconut milk has reached 105°F (41°C) add the maple syrup and your choice of starter.
8. Pour the mixture into an appropriately sized jar, cover, and place in pre-heated oven with the light left on inside as per the previous method.
9. Allow to culture 12–48 hours. Check after 12 hours. Watch for bubbles in the mixture and taste for sourness.

Notes

Important These processes are for creating your starter batch of kefir. Once your starter kefir is ready, you can then use this culture to start new batches of coconut kefir, and you can reduce the amount of maple syrup or other sweetener.

Sweeteners that you can use to feed your culture as it adjusts to coconut milk are: maple syrup, raw agave, raw sugar, raw cane juice crystals, and white sugar (not my preference). Stevia is not a suitable food source for the culture.

The starter batch may come out stronger than you anticipate; the goal of this is to produce a large amount of probiotic which can then be used to culture subsequent batches.

Storing coconut kefir culture After the culturing process, the coconut kefir should be stored covered in the refrigerator. Providing that the jar has been properly sanitized and that there has been no cross-contamination, the coconut kefir can stay covered in the refrigerator for up to 3 weeks.

Using the Starter Batch for Subsequent Batches

Now that you've made your starter batch (from which you make subsequent batches of kefir), here is the method for a larger batch of coconut kefir. Since the goal is not to produce kefir grains in and of themselves, but to produce a curd, or more firm mass (thicker than yogurt, almost solid), it is indeed possible to use the whey or fluid from one batch to start the next.

You can choose between either of the processes (not pre-heating the coconut milk or pre-heating it) to make your batch of coconut kefir curd.

I use both methods of making coconut kefir depending on what I am trying to achieve in the way of the cheese's taste and texture.

I use the pre-heated coconut milk method in conjunction with a longer culturing time period when I want to make a fresh, bright-tasting cheese with a creamy texture that will age well into a firmer, more crumbly feta-like texture. I use the mesophilic, or 100°F (38°C) method (no pre-heating of the coconut milk), when I am seeking to make a sour cream, yogurt, or very soft cheese curd.

PROBIOTIC CAPSULES, MISO, TEMPEH CULTURE, SAUERKRAUT BRINE

This section outlines some of the plant-based culturing mediums which can be used directly, without having to be fed or trained onto mediums prior to use.

Probiotic capsules These can be found in a number of health food stores, natural food supply shops, and even mainstream pharmacies and grocery stores. Be sure to read the labels closely to ensure that the capsules are not made of gelatine, and are labelled vegan friendly.

Probiotic capsules are used by many people to aid with digestion. They consist of a mixture of bacteria that are naturally found within our gut. These bacteria assist us in digesting a variety of foods, process nutrients that we would not otherwise easily obtain, and through such interactions assist the delivery of nutrients to the rest of our bodies.

These bacteria feed on carbohydrates just as we do, and in the process alter their feeding medium. Fruit juice becomes wine, mashed barley and hops become beer, wine becomes vinegar. Kombucha, ginger beer, yogurt, dairy-based cheese, sourdough bread and many other foods derive their flavors from the process of bacteria (and also, in these examples, yeasts) acting on a medium.

Using probiotics in culturing plant-based cheese has been an active pursuit of many people for several years. Matthew Kenney of the renowned Matthew Kenney Culinary Academy (a plant-based gourmet culinary institute), teaches basic culturing classes in his program. Many holistic nutritionists and raw food culinarians also teach basic cultured nut-based cheese classes using probiotics in the culturing process.

Miso A fermented paste made from soybeans, brown rice, barley, and other legumes (there is a great chickpea miso sold in Canada by Feeding Change), miso is fermented using the fungi *aspergillus oryzae,* and is a staple food item in Japanese cuisine.

As a probiotic-rich paste with a great deal of umami, miso presents an interesting and useful culturing agent for plant-based cheeses. It can be used alone for the umami effect in flavoring non-cultured cheezes but I also like to use it to culture a nut-or seed-based mixture.

Two recipes in the following chapter include miso as an active culturing agent.

Sauerkraut brine Sauerkraut has long been understood as a digestive aid, and has seen a resurgence of popularity with the increasing awareness of its nutritional benefits and ease of making.

Sauerkraut brine (the fluid in which sauerkraut is stored) is full of lactobacilli and naturally occurring yeasts. It is very tangy and will certainly culture a nut or seed base, but it will also impart a subtle cabbage flavor.

While this may not be everyone's preferred flavor, if used with cultured cheeses to which you plan to add other stronger flavors, it could work well. I have enjoyed testing a variety of nuts and seeds, and find that sauerkraut brine can work very well with cashews, sunflower seeds, and macadamia nuts. I would avoid using it with almonds, as almond and cabbage both have a lot of sulfur compounds and this could lead to a rather strong odor and somewhat unpleasant flavor.

Tempeh culture I have only begun experimenting with tempeh starter culture as a plant-based cheese culture. Tempeh is a traditional Indonesian food—fermented soy pressed into a cake. When used as a starter, the culture may be fed on soy, but does not carry with it soy flavor or a meaningful amount of soy content. Thus far in my experiments, I have found tempeh culture does create a nice umami flavor with pumpkin seeds, sunflower seeds, and in two legume cheese tests I have been working on with chickpeas and lentils.

The next chapter does not include recipes or methods for using sauerkraut brine and tempeh cultures, However, I do think it is worth exploring further the culturing ability of both of them. I have begun testing both as secondary culturing agents on some of my cheeses, using them for washing rinds or for adding to a mixture after a primary stage of culturing. I encourage you to try them for yourself.

5

FRESH CULTURED CHEESES

THIS CHAPTER PRESENTS several recipes for cultured cheeses that are easy to make and take very little time. They will still take more time than one of the cheezes, but it is worth the small amount of waiting time for the cultures to do their work!

These cheeses mirror their dairy-based versions to the extent that they are shorter-term cultured cheeses, soft, and typically made with a single culturing aid. Texturally, these will be somewhat familiar to those who are nostalgic for dairy cheese, but not perfectly so. They do, however, begin to truly demonstrate that plant-based cheese can indeed be a "thing," despite the hard and fast definition of the Codex Alimentarius.

ALMOND RICOTTA

This is one of my favorite quick-cultured cheeses to make. I use a number of different nuts and seeds based on what I feel like making for a particular purpose. The recipe below uses almonds.

Method

1. Soak the almonds 1 hour to overnight in filtered water. Use a little hot water to help during the peeling process. Peel almonds.
2. In a high-speed blender, add the water, salt, and then almonds.
3. Start at low speed, then gradually increase speed. Blend until smooth.
4. Pour the mixture into a cheesecloth bag and allow to drain from 4 hours to overnight.
5. Remove the drained mixture into a clean, sanitized food-grade plastic container or bowl. Break open the capsule of probiotic and add. Gently stir into the mixture.
6. Cover tightly, and allow to culture at room temperature overnight. This ricotta only needs to culture for 8–12 hours. Up to 15 hours or a bit longer is fine, if you like a stronger flavor.

Note If your kitchen is very warm (above 77°F [25°C]), place the container in the fridge. It will take longer but it will still culture.

As the mixture cultures, make notes on what you observe. You should see bubbles forming, and the mixture looking fluffy and aerated. You will see some whey or fluid formation at the bottom of the container as the ricotta moves to the surface.

After the ricotta has cultured, pour the mixture into a cheesecloth or nut milk bag and strain off the whey. You can save the whey and use it to start a new batch, but make sure to keep this in a sealed jar and refrigerated, and only for up to 2 weeks. Remove the ricotta from the bag and taste again. You can add other components, such as garlic or garlic powder, lemon, herbs, or dried fruit. Store in a sealed container for up to 2 weeks in the refrigerator.

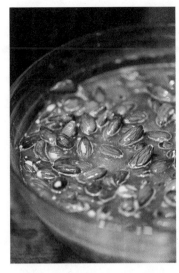

▲ Soaking almonds.
CATHERINE DOWNES

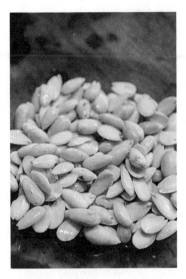

▲ Peeled almonds.
CATHERINE DOWNES

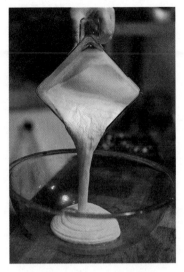

▲ Blended almond base for
making cultured almond ricotta.
CATHERINE DOWNES

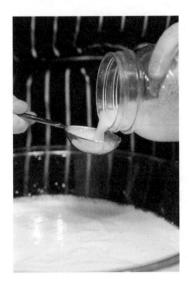

▲ Adding coconut kefir as
culturing agent to almond
base. CATHERINE DOWNES

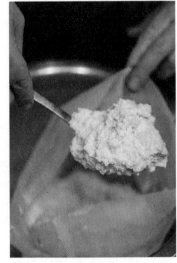

▲ Cultured almond ricotta
after culturing and draining.
CATHERINE DOWNES

QUESO FRESCO

EQUIPMENT

High-speed blender

Spatula

Container for culturing

Cheesecloth

Measuring cups

Measuring spoons

INGREDIENTS

3 cups cashews, macadamia
nuts, or combination
of the two, soaked from
1 hour to overnight.

2–3 tsp salt

1½ cups filtered water,
plus more for blending
as needed

1 probiotic capsule, or
⅛ cup coconut kefir
or ⅛ cup rejuvelac

½ cup full-fat coconut milk
(optional)

Traditionally, queso fresco is a Mexican cheese made from raw cow or goat milk. Literally it means "fresh cheese." The cheese is soft to semi-soft but not liquidy. Many plant-based quesos apply the term very loosely. As the intent of this book is to honor the craft of cheesemaking in general and identify how plant-based cheesemaking can legitimately be viewed as an evolution of cheesemaking itself, I am offering a recipe that should yield a thicker, more naturally tangy cheese than some of the other plant-based versions.

Probiotic choice: Whether you use the probiotic capsule, the coconut kefir, or the rejuvelac is up to you. Each one will create slightly different flavors and intensity, so it becomes a matter of preference. A strong rejuvelac cultures very quickly, so if you use it, you may want to reduce the maximum culturing time. Tasting every few hours during the culturing process will allow you to best determine what you enjoy the most.

Method

1. Add the water (coconut milk if you use it), salt, and nuts to a high-speed blender.

2. Starting on low speed, and gradually working up to higher speed, stop and periodically scrape the mixture down the sides of the blender pitcher. If it is too thick and binding around the blender blades, add small amounts of filtered water and blend at low to moderate speed until the mixture is very smooth.

3. Scrape the mixture into a clean, sanitized container. Add the probiotic capsule or the coconut kefir culture. Cover and allow to culture at room temperature up to 24 hours. Check after 12 hours.

4. You should observe bubble activity (evidence the culture is happy and healthy) and upon tasting find it mildly to moderately tangy.

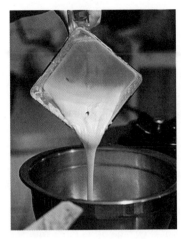

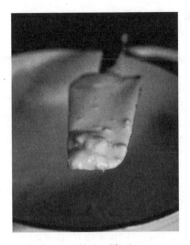

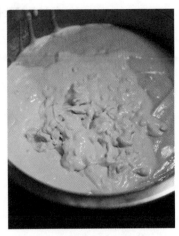

▲ Texture of blended cashew medium for making queso fresco prior to adding culture. CATHERINE DOWNES

▲ Cashew curd being lifted on spoon. CATHERINE DOWNES

▲ Cashew curd for cashew queso fresco before draining in cheese-cloth. CATHERINE DOWNES

5. After it has cultured to the strength you like, put the mixture into a cheesecloth bag or nut milk bag, and allow to drain for from 4 hours to overnight, depending on how firm you want the cheese to be.

6. After draining, you can choose to keep the cheese as is and store in a clean, sanitized covered container in the refrigerator. This can keep for up to 30 days, but may become a little stronger in flavor over the course of time.

7. You can also form the cheese. Using your choice of form, for instance a timbale (circular form without a bottom), press the cheese into the form and allow it to sit on a wooden board in the refrigerator for a day or two. This will allow a bit more moisture to evaporate, and you will end up with a slightly firmer cheese, which is very nice for presentation.

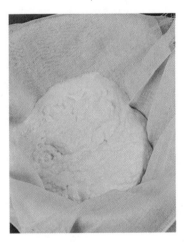

▲ Cashew queso fresco draining in cheesecloth. COLIN MEDHURST

The flavor should be lightly salty, and mildly to moderately tangy. It should have a creamy mouth feel, and hold together when picked up with your fingers.

This cheese can be used on vegan tacos, bruschetta, flat breads, salads, and, as always, anyway you like it. You can also consider adding herbs, garlic, or other seasonings.

CHEVRE STYLE

EQUIPMENT

High-speed blender

Spatula

Food-grade plastic bowl
    or container

Container to store cheese

Doubled-up cheesecloth
    or butter muslin

INGREDIENTS

3 cups cashews, macadamia
    nuts, or combination
    of the two, soaked from
    1 hour to overnight.

1–2 tsp salt

1½ cups filtered water plus
    more for blending (do
    not add all at one time)

⅛ cup coconut kefir or
    ⅛ cup rejuvelac or
    1 probiotic capsule

½ cup full-fat coconut milk
    (optional)

Note if you choose to use
    the full-fat coconut milk,
    you will need to reduce
    the amount of water.

Chevre, a style of cheese made traditionally with goat's milk, is noted for its particular tangy, sour nature, soft mouth feel, and creaminess. It is not a hard or even semi-soft cheese, but is a shaped cheese, usually seen in long rolls.

This recipe differs very slightly in culturing duration from the previous one. The longer a mixture cultures, the more of the sugars are consumed, the tangier or sharper it tastes, and the more moisture is removed from it as a by-product. The yield in longer-aged cheeses is lower than with fresher cheeses, but the trade off is more intense flavor and firmer texture.

Method

1. Add the cashew/macadamia and salt to the blender, add a little water at a time (not all at once). If you choose to use the full-fat coconut milk, also add small amounts at a time.

2. Start on low speed and gradually work up to higher speed, stopping to periodically scrape the mixture down the sides of the blender. If it's too thick and binding around the blender blades, add small amounts of filtered water and blend at low to moderate speed until the mixture is very smooth. It is really important to start the blending process on low speed. It will save your blender blades, and it will yield a smoother paste.

3. Scrape the mixture into a clean and sanitized container. Add the coconut kefir, rejuvelac culture, or probiotic capsule. Cover and allow to culture in a warm environment. If your kitchen is warm, (over 68°F [20°C]) you can do this by setting your culturing mixture near the warmest area of your kitchen, such as near your oven. You can also pre-heat your oven to 100°F (38°C), turn the heat off and — leaving the oven light on — place the covered culturing mixture inside the oven to culture temperature up to 36 hours. Check after 12 hours.

4. It is important to taste the mixture when you check it, because this is how, in part, you will know if the culture is working. The mixture should taste tangy, almost sour, a little like yogurt or sour cream. You should also check the mixture visually. You should see some bubbles — this is an indication that the cultures are working.

5. After it has cultured to the strength that you like, put the mixture into a cheesecloth bag or nut milk bag, and allow to drain from 4 hours to overnight, depending on how firm you want the cheese to be. If you allow to drain overnight, be sure to do so in the refrigerator.

6. After draining, you can keep the cheese as is and store in a clean, sanitized, covered container in the refrigerator. Because you are using live cultures, periodically remove the cover and allow gasses, the by-product of culturing, to escape. This can keep for up to 14 days, but may become a little stronger in flavor over the course of time. This will be a soft, fresh cheese.

7. The flavor should be lightly salty, and tangy. It should have a creamy mouth feel, and hold together when picked up with your fingers. Below are some modifications that you can use to create different flavors.

Modifications

Truffle and black pepper

You can use either white or black truffle oil (2 tsp will be sufficient), or, if you have deep pockets, you can shave fresh truffle.

Add 1–2 tsp coarse black or pink peppercorn (preferably cracked with mortar and pestle or pepper grinder — this will yield a clean and fresh pepper flavor).

Add both the truffle element and the peppercorn after the culturing process has been completed. Fold it into the mixture, then form the cheeses.

Fig and cassis

Add ⅛ cup very finely diced dried fig at the time of blending and culture it along with the rest of the mixture. This will add a mildly

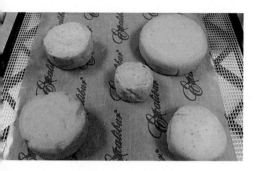

▲ Sample of cheese drying (1).
AUTHOR

wine-type flavor. After culturing add another ⅛ cup of chopped fig. This will add a sweeter fig flavor and finally add 1 tbsp cassis. This will give the cheese a decadent feel.

Note If you make this modification, air-drying the cheese will yield a better result than putting the cheese into a covered container right away. The dried fruit will add its own natural yeasts to the culturing process, so, if covered, they will be encouraged to grow. If you air-dry the cheese a bit, the excess gasses of culturing will evaporate, and the flavor will develop more complexity.

Herb and Garlic

After the culturing and draining process, add 1 tbsp finely minced chives, 1 tbsp minced fresh tarragon, ½ tbsp minced fresh rosemary, and ½ tbsp garlic powder or 1 tbsp finely minced fresh garlic. You can also add less herb if you wish; this modification is merely a suggestion.

Forming and Aging

This particular cheese can be served young (after 48 hours of culturing) or can be dry-aged. I'll discuss other cheese aging and rind curing processes in more detail further on; however, this is how you can age this particular cheese and allow it to develop a more complex flavor and texture with or without the amendments above.

1. Once the initial culturing and draining has occurred, shape the cheese into logs or other shapes as you wish. Do this after you add other elements if using one of the above amendments.
2. Wrap the cheese in cheesecloth or butter muslin and place on bamboo mats on top of wood or bamboo boards. Cheesecloth and wood absorb moisture. Evaporation of moisture is essential in the aging of cheeses, as it allows them to last longer.
3. Place the board into the refrigerator making sure there is nothing that will touch the cheeses. Do not cover; rather, leave the cheese

exposed to the cool air. This will further remove moisture. I often use the vegetable drawer in my fridge in order to keep the cheese away from other items in the fridge.

4. Allow this dry-aging to occur for up to 2 days. Check both taste and texture daily. Dry-aged cheese will keep longer than most of the fresh cheeses or cheeze, up to 30 days in ideal conditions. After the cheese has dry-aged, keep it wrapped tightly in plastic wrap, and stored in the refrigerator.

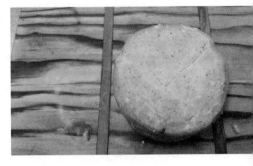

▲ Sample of cheese drying (2).
AUTHOR

SHORT-AGED AND SEMI-SOFT CHEESES

Again, the classification system I am employing is solely mine, and primarily one I use to help me understand the processes I am working and experimenting with. There is nothing like working with live cultures to teach you that you know very little about many things. The world of microbes is a fascinating one that is integrally tied with human evolution.

The short-aged and semi-soft cheeses I refer to here generally use a kefir-based culture (coconut, water, or otherwise nut-based). I work a lot with coconut and water kefir and so I'll refer primarily to these starter cultures within the recipes and processes provided. I particularly enjoy the level of acidity healthy and happy kefir cultures provide, and find that they allow the cheeses to age well. However, the methods described here can be used with other lactic acid-producing cultures such as rejuvelac or probiotic capsules.

While these cheeses will not have all the characteristics of dairy-based cheeses, my goal is to present something that can be understood as a new form of cheese in its own right, rather than attempting to copy or mimic traditional dairy cheeses.

Below I detail three types of kefir curd that I commonly use for making short-aged and semi-soft plant-based cheeses. They can all be used as young, fresh cheeses, or as the bases for short to longer-aged cheeses, or cheeses to which secondary cultures are added.

COCONUT KEFIR CURD

EQUIPMENT

Stainless steel stock pot

Food-grade plastic or glass
     bowl/bucket

Large spoon

Spatula

Cheesecloth or butter
     muslin

Bamboo mat

Wood board

Cheese mold (optional)

INGREDIENTS

1 L coconut milk, full fat

⅛ cup coconut kefir starter
     (from previous starter
     batch)

½ tbsp maple syrup

1 tsp salt added (after
     draining, and before
     molding/shaping)

While you can use this method and culture for shorter periods of time to end up with a drinkable kefir or slightly thicker yogurt, the object of the process is to end up with a thick, well-coagulated curd. The development of a curd relies on longer culturing time and you may want to add a sweetener (maple syrup, agave, coconut sugar), which slows down the rate of culturing and therefore allows flavor to develop without becoming too "sour"/acidic too quickly. The resulting curd can then be used to mix with other nut-based pastes or on its own.

The following recipe is designed to provide you with some working curd to do with as you wish.

Method

To make the coconut kefir curd you may either choose to pre-heat (pasteurize) your coconut milk, or to culture it without pre-heating first. If you choose to pre-heat your coconut milk, be sure to follow the instructions for bringing it to temperature and for cooling prior to adding the kefir starter culture in order to avoid killing the culture. If you add culture at too high a temperature (above 180°F [82°C]), you risk killing the bacteria and yeasts which you need to create the level of acidity required to make the kefir curd.

If you choose to culture without pasteurizing the coconut milk first, you will have to be particularly attentive to maintaining a consistent culturing temperature, and checking the mixture as it cultures.

After you decide whether to pasteurize your coconut milk or not, refer to the section on making your starter culture for the pasteurization process. If you are not pasteurizing, you can place the coconut milk in the refrigerator for a couple of hours first to separate coconut water from the fat, and then strain off the water. This is not necessary, as you can culture the coconut milk as is and then strain the excess

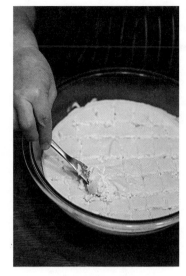

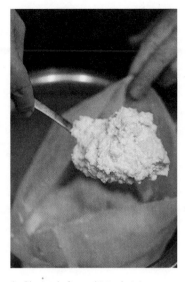

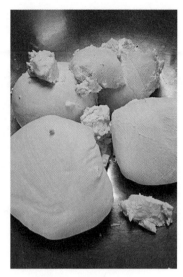

▲ Kefir curd. CATHERINE DOWNES   ▲ Placing kefir curd into draining   ▲ Kefir curd balls. AUTHOR
bag. CATHERINE DOWNES

fluid after the curd is formed, but if you want to remove a lot of excess
moisture earlier on, this will certainly help to yield a thicker curd.

Culturing Method

1. Place your coconut milk (pasteurized or un-pasteurized) into a food-
    grade plastic container, glass bowl, or jar.

2. Add the starter culture to the coconut milk and the sweetener, cover
    the top of the jar, bucket, or bowl, and maintain a culturing tempera-
    ture between 68–105°F (20–40°C) for 12–48 hours. If you have a
    yogurt maker or a slow cooker that can maintain this low a heat, you
    can use them for this purpose.

3. Alternatively, you can use your oven to maintain the culturing tem-
    perature: pre-heat the oven to 100°F (38°C) for 30 minutes, then turn
    the heat off and leave the oven light on to provide a suitable tempera-
    ture for culturing. Just make sure that the oven is clean, and that
    the culturing container is well covered. Alternatively, you can use
    a yogurt maker to maintain the culturing temperature.

4. Check the kefir every 12 hours. Taste a small amount to check the acidity in terms of flavor or use pH testing strips. Acidity should be 4.6 pH or lower. If the kefir is not starting to taste sour, discard and start again. You should also be able to see bubbles which are signs that the culturing bacteria are active.

5. After the curd is finished culturing, strain it through cheesecloth/nut milk bag for 4 hours to overnight. After draining, the curd should be soft but clump together. You can use it is as a soft cheese, or follow the modifications in the previous section and make a flavored softer cheese. For instructions on dry-aging the cheese see Chapter 6.

6. You can also use this curd to mix with cashew, macadamia, or almond paste to culture a new cheese. I often combine coconut kefir curd with almond paste to make an aged cheddar-style cheese.

Note If you do not have access to water kefir grains or coconut kefir culture, but do have a friend with dairy-fed grain or are open to using a small amount of dairy-based kefir to start your first batch, remember that the "grains," as they are called, are actually bacteria and yeast, and breed very quickly.

If you do make a starter batch using this last method, strain the grain out of the fluid portion, discard the fluid portion, and place the grains with a bit of maple syrup into another batch of coconut milk. This trains the kefir grain onto a new feeding medium. After this batch they are fully plant-based friendly.

CULTURED CASHEW
KEFIR CURD

Method

1. Soak cashews overnight in filtered water then drain.

2. Place all ingredients except the culturing agent in a high-speed blender.

3. Start at low speed and progress slowly to high speed, adding small amounts of filtered water and blending until consistency is smooth and creamy.

4. Pour the mixture into a glass or non-metallic bowl. Pour in your choice of culturing agent (kefir is preferred, but you can use a probiotic capsule or rejuvelac) and stir together well.

5. Cover the top of the bowl tightly with cling wrap. Place in the pre-heated oven and allow to culture for 12–48 hours.

> **INGREDIENTS**
>
> 3 cups cashews, soaked
> overnight
> 1½ tsp salt
> ¼ cup coconut kefir, water
> kefir, or rejuvelac starter
> 2 cups filtered water
> ½ tbsp maple syrup

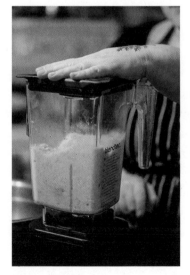

▲ Cashews blending.
CATHERINE DOWNES

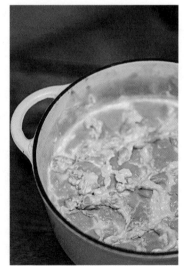

▲ Cashew curd.
CATHERINE DOWNES

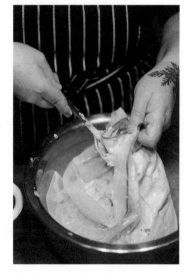

▲ Placing cashew curd into draining bag. CATHERINE DOWNES

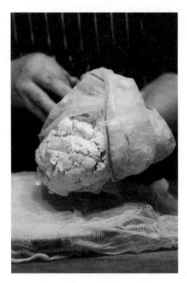

▲ Removing cashew curd from draining bag. CATHERINE DOWNES

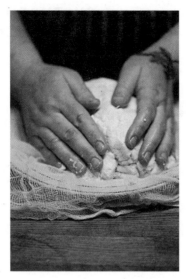

▲ Forming curd in cheesecloth wrap. CATHERINE DOWNES

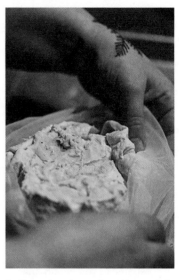

▲ Removing cheese from cheesecloth. CATHERINE DOWNES

6. Check the curd after 12 hours and run a clean knife through it to test its consistency. Taste a small amount to check for acidity. Observe it for bubbles, the sign that the culture is active. Cover the top of the bowl again and leave to culture. Check every 6–12 hours. If at any point before the 48 hours is up, you find the mixture to be too sour, stop culturing and refrigerate. You can still use it either as a sour cream to thicken sauces, or sweeten it to make it more like a yogurt. Keep in mind that for the most part "too sour" is a personal preference and not a sign that the mixture is off.

7. After the culturing process is finished, pour the mixture into a cheesecloth or nut milk bag. Allow to drain for 2 hours to overnight.

8. After you have finished draining the curd, you can use it as is, or add other flavors and use it as a cream cheese or crème fraîche of sorts. Alternatively, you can then place the curd into cheesecloth- or butter muslin-lined molds and press the curd to make a firmer cheese. For further instructions on turning your curd into a firmer cheese, see Chapter 6.

CULTURED ALMOND CURD

I use almond curd in several of my Blue Heron cheeses, particularly for those cheeses that I wish to age for longer periods of time. The sulfur content of the almonds seems to allow the curd to age nicely into a sharp, tangy flavor as the cheese ages. In my efforts, I have found the cheese to be a bit reminiscent of a cheddar, and on occasion to smell and taste mildly of mushroom. The almond curd allows for some interesting and complex flavors to develop. Almond curd can be a bit finicky when cultured, as it can become too sour relatively quickly, which will make it seem off and unpalatable to eat on its own at that stage. It is, however, at this point that the curd can be further air-dried, salted, and aged to become a firmer, stronger tasting cheese.

If you choose to experiment with an almond curd that may have gone too far, ensure that it is not contaminated by other microbes before doing so. If other growths (red mold, black mold and such) are present, discard and start again.

> **INGREDIENTS**
> 3 cups almonds, soaked
> 3 tsp salt
> 1–2 tbsp maple syrup
> ¼ cup coconut kefir culture
> (you can use rejuvelac
> here, but use ⅛ cup
> instead)
> 3–4 cups of water

Method

1. Soak almonds in warm to almost hot water for about 1 hour then peel the skins off. (Removing the skins is much easier with warmer water.)

2. Add all of the ingredients, beginning with the water and excluding the culturing agent, to a high-speed blender.

3. Start on low speed and progress to higher speed, stopping periodically to scrape down the sides of the pitcher. Starting slow cannot be overemphasized. Almonds, even when soaked, are quite hard, and can take a toll on your blender blades. I often pulse for several minutes or grind the almonds in a food processor first before blending them into a nut milk/nut paste.

4. Once the mixture is thick and creamy, pour into a glass or food-grade plastic bowl and pour in the culturing agent. Cover the top of

the bowl with cling wrap and place in an oven pre-heated to 100°F (38°C) and allow to culture for 12–36 hours.

5. Check the mixture after 12 hours, taste for sourness, observe for bubbles and a slightly fluffy appearance. There should also be some whey (fluid that has separated from the mixture). The presence of the maple syrup will allow the mixture to culture longer, avoiding some of the harsh tanginess that can occur with almonds. You will not need to culture the almond mixture past the 12 hours.

6. After the mixture has finished culturing, pour into a cheesecloth or nut milk bag and allow to drain from 2 hours to overnight. If draining overnight, be sure to place in the refrigerator.

Store the curd in a sealed container and save for using to make cheese. Keeps for up to 2 weeks, refrigerated.

COCONUT KEFIR AND
MACADAMIA GARLIC AND HERB CHEESE

Method

1. Soak the macadamia nuts overnight.
2. In a high-speed blender add half the water and all the macadamia nuts.
3. Start on low speed, progressing gradually to high speed. Blend the nuts until very smooth. Add the lemon juice, salt, garlic, and more water if needed.
4. When blended completely scrape from the pitcher into a bowl then add the herbs and the coconut kefir. Stir and fold the mixture together. Place in a cheesecloth or nut milk bag, and allow to drain for up to 4 hours.
5. Using a springform pan (6–8 inch) on a wood board (so you won't need the pan bottom), place a large square of cheesecloth in the pan, large enough to cover the bottom and fall over the sides of the pan. Pour the cheese mixture into the cheesecloth and use an offset spatula or washed and sanitized hands to press the curd into place in the form. Fold the cheesecloth over, place in a cool area of your kitchen (below 68°F [20°C]), and cover the top of the pan with plastic wrap. Leave at room temperature for up to 4 hours. This will allow the kefir curd to culture the macadamia a little.
6. Keep the cheese covered and place the set up in your refrigerator. Allow to culture at low temperature in the refrigerator for 2 days, then remove the plastic. Fold back the cheesecloth and sprinkle a little salt over the top of the cheese. Remove the springform and lay out some clean cheesecloth. Gently lift the cheese onto the new cheesecloth and slip the older cheesecloth off. Flip the cheese gently and sprinkle salt over the bottom and sides as well. The salting of the rind helps excess moisture come to the surface and then evaporate. At this time, you may also choose to cover the rind in a mixture of crushed, dried herbs.

> **INGREDIENTS**
>
> 2 cups macadamia nuts, soaked
> 2 cups coconut kefir curd (as per recipe/method above)
> 2 tsp salt
> ⅛ cup lemon juice
> 2 tsp garlic powder or 1½ tbsp minced fresh garlic
> 2 tbsp herbs of your choice (I like to use rosemary, dill, tarragon), fresh, minced (or 3 tbsp dried herbs)
> 1 cup filtered water for blending

7. Check the cheese every day and flip it over, changing the wood board if needed. As the cheese loses moisture it will firm up. After the first day, however, you can eat it.

8. The longer this cheese air dries, the longer it keeps. This cheese ages quite well, and whether you choose to eat it soft, or firmer and more crumbly is up to you. After you have aged it to the hardness you like (I recommend no more than 7 days), wrap tightly in plastic wrap or cheese paper and refrigerate. It should keep for up to 30 days.

Note This cheese undergoes a very minor secondary culturing process when the cheese is left covered at room temperature for 4 hours after the inclusion of the macadamia paste, as the cultures in the mixture will then begin culturing the macadamia paste.

An alternative possibility here is that you can blend the macadamia paste first, without the other ingredients, mix it with the coconut kefir curd, and allow that mixture to culture together for 12–24 hours (covered, and in an oven pre-heated to 100°F [38°C], heat off, light left on).

FETA-STYLE CHEESES

I am including two feta-type recipes, as each is very different from the other, and allows you to practice using different culturing mediums, yielding very different flavor profiles.

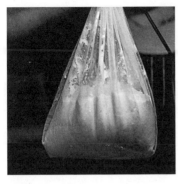

▲ Kefir/cheese curd draining. CATHERINE DOWNES

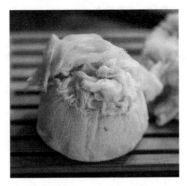

▲ Kefir/macadamia cheese in cheesecloth. CATHERINE DOWNES

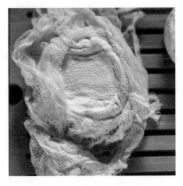

▲ Partially unwrapped kefir macadamia cheese. CATHERINE DOWNES

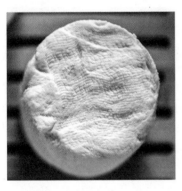

▲ Kefir/macadamia cheese fully unwrapped and aging.
CATHERINE DOWNES

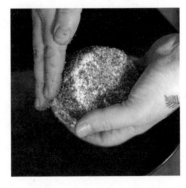

▲ Kefir/macadamia cheese being herb rinded. CATHERINE DOWNES

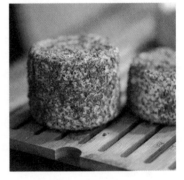

▲ Herbed kefir/macadamia cheese dry aging on wood rack. CATHERINE DOWNES

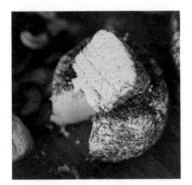

▲ Herbed kefir/macadamia cheese with wedge cut out. CATHERINE DOWNES

COCONUT KEFIR FETA

INGREDIENTS

4 cups coconut kefir curd
(see instructions above
for making coconut
kefir curd)

1 tbsp salt

Method

1. Mix the salt and coconut kefir together. Place in a fine mesh bag (such as the vegetable bags you find in Whole Foods or brewing supply stores). I recommend doubling up the bags. Allow to drain for up to 12 hours. The salt will help to remove moisture.

2. Cut 2 pieces of cheesecloth into approximately 12 inches by the width of your cloth. Divide the cheese into two even-sized sections. Place each section on a piece of cheesecloth. Fold each cheese into a well-wrapped package. Place the cheese packages on a wood board and set in the refrigerator but do not cover with plastic.

3. The cheesecloth will help in moisture evaporation. After 2 days, unwrap the cheeses and sprinkle some very fine salt over the surface, and rewrap in fresh cheesecloth. You will also want to change the board as it will have absorbed moisture.

4. Place the rewrapped cheeses back into the fridge, and repeat this process every 2 days for up to 10 days. As you salt and rewrap the cheese, you should find that it gets firmer and drier. Once it is very firm to touch, remove the cheese from the fridge and cut into 2 cm. cubes (or whatever size you like).

5. If the cheese is dry and firm enough you can consider storing it in olive oil with herbs in a sealed container in the refrigerator for up to 30 days, but be sure to check for quality of flavor, and make sure the cubes are not disintegrating.

6. If it is still soft, continue to air dry the cubes until they are quite firm. They can then be stored in a sealed container and kept for up to 2 weeks.

Note I have experimented with keeping the very dry feta kefir in a light brine water (2 tbsp salt to 2 L water), but eventually the cheese will erode in the salt water because the cheese doesn't have the same protein structure as dairy-based feta. I have had more success storing the cheese in sunflower oil.

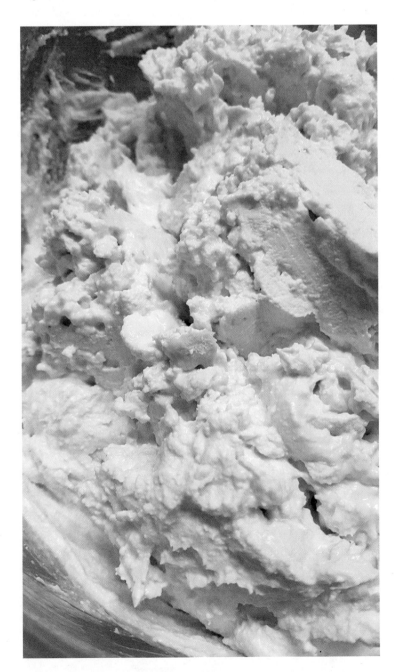

◀ Coconut kefir feta at curd stage.
AUTHOR

ALMOND CURD FETA

INGREDIENTS

3 cups almond kefir curd
  (see instructions for
  almond kefir curd above)
Filtered water for blending
  (use only small amounts
  at a time)
1½ tbsp salt
1 tbsp chickpea miso
½ tbsp apple cider vinegar
  or lemon juice

Method

1. Place the almond curd, salt, miso, and vinegar or lemon juice in the blender, and blend until well combined. Add small amounts of water to assist with blending if necessary. You may also use coconut milk for this purpose.

2. Starting on low speed, progress to high speed slowly, stopping and periodically scraping the mixture down the sides and continuing to blend, adding just a little water at a time to make a smooth, creamy paste.

3. Remove the mixture from the pitcher and place into a sealable container. Allow the mixture to culture overnight at room temperature. Make sure the container is approximately twice the size in volume as the amount of cheese you are making, as almonds will culture and expand quite rapidly. The miso and apple cider vinegar both have microbes which will initiate a culturing process.

4. Check every 6–12 hours to ensure that culturing has begun. You should observe air pockets or bubbles. Pay attention to the aroma, which should start to smell a bit more umami. Taste to ensure that the flavor is not too far towards the strong end as almonds can become quite bitter when cultured too long.

5. After about 12 hours, remove the cheese curd to a cheesecloth or nut milk bag and hang, allowing to drain overnight in the refrigerator. The key to making a feta-style cheese is to remove as much moisture as possible.

6. Just as you did with the coconut kefir feta, place the cheese in cheesecloth or butter muslin after draining and shape it into a square or rectangle, wrap into a package, and place on a wood board in the refrigerator. After 12 hours, unwrap, check the cheese, and sprinkle the rind with a little salt. Change the cheesecloth wrapper every 2 days and lightly salt the surface as well. With respect to this

particular cheese, I also like to take a piece of cheesecloth and rub the exterior with apple cider vinegar to help cure the surface.

7. This cheese can take up to 2 weeks to fully age, and requires daily flipping and checking of the surface. Once the cheese is almost entirely dried out, it can be cut and stored, refrigerated in a sealed jar in seasoned olive oil, or in a light salt brine in a covered container. I made a batch once and stored it in preserved lemon and cardamom brine. It kept for six months, and didn't last long once we started using it!

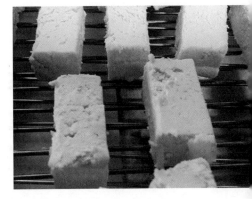

▲ Almond feta cheese test. AUTHOR

Remember that as you proceed into more advanced cheesemaking, great patience is required. Training your observational skills to recognize the right taste, texture, and appearance is not something that can be taught solely in a book or class. Books and classes are important tools, providing you with the necessary foundation of information. However, you must also train your palette, your nose, and your ability to recognize what looks and feels and tastes right, in relation to the necessary information regarding correct temperature, humidity, and pH conditions. Batches will fail, results will not always turn out as planned. Learning from failure is the only way we truly succeed.

I recommend keeping a detailed log of your cheesemaking, so that you get used to recording your observations along with dates (date made, date checked, and finished or ready). This helps to train your observations to a time frame. For instance, this will allow you to recognize if one batch is taking longer than a previous batch to become ready, or to identify which variables (temperature, humidity, pH) may need adjusting. Refer to Chapter 6 on aging methods for more tips on aging your cheeses.

6

FIRM CHEESES AND CHEESE AGING

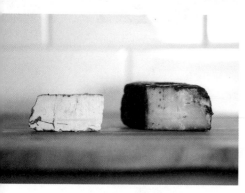

▲ Blue Heron cheeses: blue and balsamic washed-rind blue. CATHERINE DOWNES

▶ Blue Heron cheeses: black truffle cashew camembert, caraway seed mid-aged cashew-coconut gouda, and aged coconut kefir with herb. CATHERINE DOWNES

I AM DEEPLY CURIOUS about how things work, and once I began this journey of plant-based cheesemaking it seemed inevitable that I would eventually want to explore how dairy-trained cultures would interact with plant-based media. My initial foray was training dairy-fed kefir grain onto coconut and nut-based mediums; I am currently working on training a number of cultures typically used in dairy cheesemaking onto plant-based mediums with the objective of replicating them on these new mediums. So far, in testing, there has been reliable success.

In this chapter I provide two recipes for longer-aging cheeses: a gouda/havarti style and a double-cultured cheddar style as well as more detailed information and processes for aging these cheeses or even some of the other cheeses in this book. I evolved or adapted both processes in developing a variety of plant-based cheese for Blue Heron Creamery, my plant-based, dairy-free cheese company.

These processes are much more involved and require a great deal of attention to detail and timing. As with all of the recipes in this book, before you start on any recipe you *must* clean and sanitize all of your tools and work spaces.

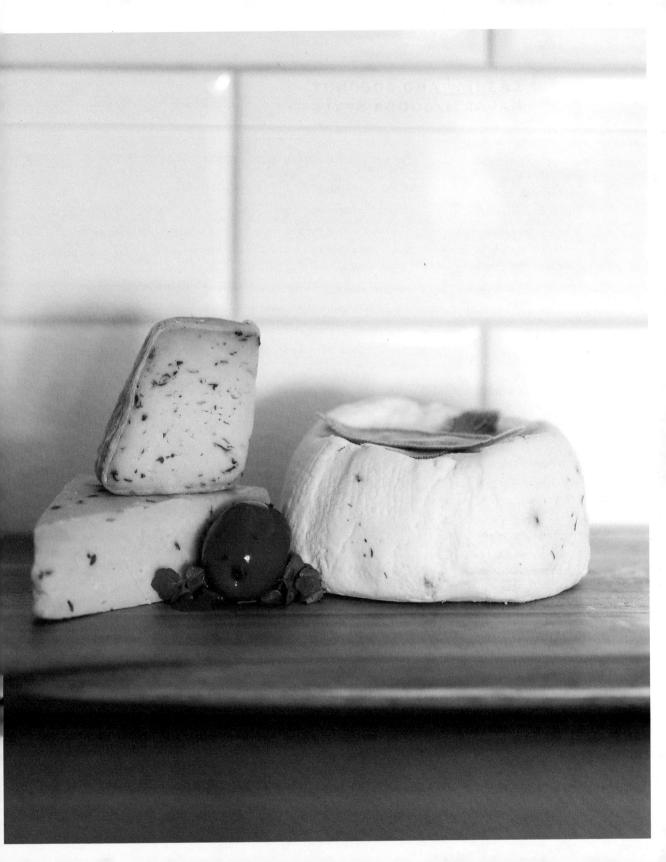

CASHEW AND COCONUT
HAVARTI/GOUDA STYLE

INGREDIENTS

3 cups cashews, soaked
for up to 2 days. This
encourages a little wild
fermentation. Change
the water every day.

1 L filtered water

2 cups coconut milk, full fat

3 tbsp apple cider vinegar
(this has live culture in
it and serves as a coagu-
lating agent).

¼ tsp vegetable rennet,
dissolved in 25 ml water

⅛ tsp mesophilic direct-set
culture (obtained from
a cheesemaking supply
shop, and optional in
this recipe)

If you elect to not use the
mesophilic direct-set
culture, you can use a
probiotic capsule or ¼
cup coconut kefir curd
or culture.

2 tsp salt

spices or herbs of your
choice: caraway, cumin,
fennel, saffron

Method

1. Clean and sanitize all equipment and surfaces.
2. Drain the cashews — they should feel quite soft. Don't be alarmed if the water may have had some bubbles, cashews like to ferment.
3. Place the cashews and ½ L of the filtered water into a high-speed blender and blend until very, very smooth. Add the apple cider vinegar and continue blending.
4. Pour the mixture into a bowl and whisk in the coconut milk.
5. Take two 6 L pots and make a water bath. Place the cashew and coconut milk mixture into the pot and gently heat the mixture to 86°F (30°C).
6. While this is heating, boil some water and in a separate bowl pour it over any spices you may choose to use. This sterilizes the seed of any wild yeast and bacteria.

   If using the mesophilic direct-set culture, dissolve in ½ cup filtered water.

   If using the coconut kefir culture instead, add directly to the mixture and whisk, maintaining low heat, keep covered, and allow to culture overnight.

   If using the 2 probiotic capsules to culture, do the same as with the coconut kefir culture.

Note Each of the above starter cultures will behave somewhat differently, but all will fulfill the goal of acidification, the first stage of culturing.

1. Dissolve the vegetable rennet in ⅛ cup water. Add the culture and the spices to the mixture and check the temperature, ensuring that it remains at 86°F (30°C).
2. Add the vegetable rennet to the mixture and stir for up to 2 minutes. The vegetable rennet will help the mixture to coagulate. This will

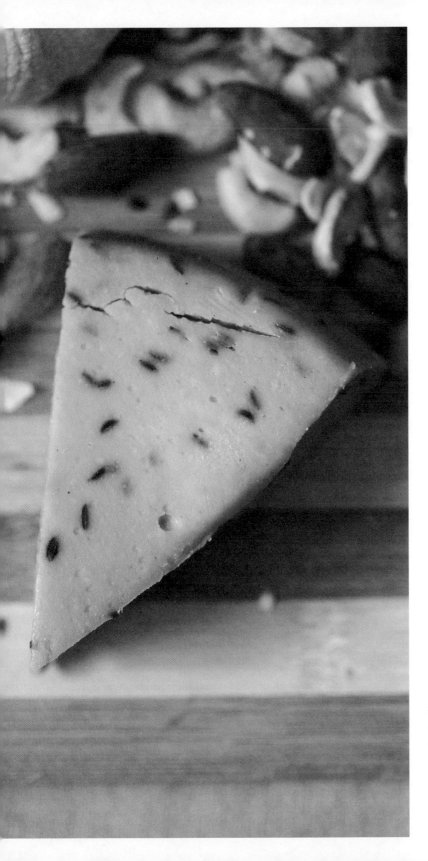

◄ Cumin seed cashew and
coconut gouda, mid-aged
(1–2 months). CATHERINE DOWNES

take up to 60 minutes if using the mesophilic direct-set culture and up to overnight if using either the coconut kefir or probiotic capsules.

3. Check the curd. It should be very thick and almost firm. This mixture will look and behave very differently than dairy curd, so if you do have dairy-based cheesemaking experience, you will not be familiar with what to look for: The curd should pull away from the sides of the pot and slicing a knife through the curd should reveal moisture (whey) at the bottom of the pot.

4. Drain the whey off into a measuring cup. Add hot tap water, equal to the amount of whey that you drained off. This in effect washes the curd, but, as this curd isn't quite the same as a dairy curd, the water will mostly mix in.

5. Warm the temperature of the water bath to 98°F (37°C) and stir the curd. Check the temperature of the mixture, and ensure that it reaches 96–98°F (36–37°C). Stir the mixture for up to 40 minutes. Ensure that the temperature neither goes below nor above this range.

   Pour the mixture into a double-layered mesh bag or doubled cheesecloth or nut milk bag, and allow to drain for up to 4 hours. Gently squeeze the bag periodically to remove excess moisture and to move the curd inside the bag.

6. Line a cheese mold (usually plastic with perforations to allow evaporation and draining) with cheesecloth and place on a sushi mat on a wood board. You can use a single large mold or several smaller ones. Place the cheese mixture into the molds and wrap the cheese over with the cheesecloth. Place the cheese on a clean wood board or bamboo mat and allow to air dry in a 40–55°F (4.5–13°C) environment (a converted wine fridge works perfectly for this). It can take up to 48 hours for the cheese surface to dry and you will need to turn the cheese 1–2 times a day during the drying process.

7. Make a saturated brine: 1 gallon water (or 3.8 L), 2 lbs salt, 1 tsp white vinegar, 1 tbsp calcium chloride (derived from limestone).

   Check the cheese — if still quite soft, change the cheesecloth and rewrap and place back in refrigerator. Check the cheese daily, and change the cheesecloth every day or every other day. Once excess moisture has begun to evaporate and the surface has begun to firm up, you can begin using the saturated brine to wash the surface of the cheese. After washing the cheese surface, place the cheese on a bamboo mat or cheese-aging mat and allow to air-dry in the refrigerator. Flip the cheese daily during air-drying.

I often consume it early, as a young gouda, but you can also elect to age it either by vacuum sealing the cheese or using cheese wax to seal the rind. Age the cheese between 55–60°F (13–15°C) for up to 4 months. A wine fridge is best for this, as you can adjust the temperature without affecting other things such as food, and keep the aging cheese away from other food items.

CASHEW AND COCONUT
DOUBLE-CULTURED "CHEDDAR"

INGREDIENTS

2 cups cashews soaked
overnight to 2 days (if
soaking past one night,
be sure to change the
water every day)

2 cups coconut kefir curd

1–2 tsp turmeric (optional,
for coloring)

1 tsp paprika (optional,
for coloring)

400 ml port wine (optional)

¼ tsp vegetable rennet
dissolved in 25 ml
filtered water

1 probiotic capsule

3 tsp salt

Miso brine (¼ container
of miso — I use chickpea
miso — 1 L water,
1 tbsp salt, 1 tbsp
white vinegar)

This cheese involves a double culturing process. The first stage of culturing uses coconut kefir and a probiotic capsule to create acidity and flavor complexity. Secondary culturing will occur through washing the rind with the miso brine.

While not a true cheddar process, which uses a stirred curd, this cheese uses a modified stirred-curd, plant-based cheddar process that will yield a familiar cheese.

Method

1. Clean and sanitize all equipment and work surfaces.
2. Use two pots to create a water bath and heat the water in the bottom pot to 88°F (31°C).
3. Drain the cashews and blend with 800 ml filtered water until creamy and smooth.
4. Add the turmeric and paprika for coloring if you desire.
5. Place the cashew mixture and the coconut kefir curd into the pot then place pot inside the water bath (sort of like a double boiler set up).
6. Add the probiotic capsule and heat the mixture to 88°F (31°C). Hold at this temperature and allow the mixture to ripen for up to 40 minutes.
7. Dilute the vegetable rennet in ⅛ cup filtered water then stir into the mixture. Allow the mixture to coagulate for at least 30 minutes.
8. Check to make sure that the curd is pulling away from side of the pot. It should be quite thick and a bit lumpy. Some of the curd will stick to the sides of the pot; just scrape it back into the mixture. Check the temperature to ensure it is still the same. Don't be concerned if the thickening process takes a while, this process can take up to 4 hours.
9. Once the curd has coagulated, use a clean knife to slice it in long strips. Whey, the cultured fluid that separates from the solid curd, will seep up. Drain off any whey that may be produced.

10. Bring the curd up to 102°F (39°C) and stir occasionally for 45 minutes. If using a pH meter, the pH should be between 6.1 and 6.2.

11. Drain the curd again (using cheesecloth and a strainer) to release any moisture, then return mixture to the pot and continue stirring it about every 5 minutes for an hour. The pH will drop to between 5.3 and 5.4.

12. If you desire, you can add 400 ml (14 ounces) of port wine, to make a port wine cheddar. If you do, stir it well into the mixture and let stand for 30 minutes. Drain liquid and strain the curds in a nut milk bag.

13. Allow the mixture to drain for up to 4 hours or up to overnight. The longer you drain the curd, the more moisture you will express, and therefore your cheese will end up firmer.

14. Pour the mixture into a cheesecloth-lined mold and press it into the mold. I like to use a bottomless springform or a cheese mold with holes that allow for continuous draining, resting them on a bamboo mat on top of a wood board for this purpose. I then place a weighted plate, or "follow" (a plastic insert that fits inside a matching mold), on top of the cheese to serve as a press. Allow the weight to compress the cheese for several hours. Change the cheesecloth and the board after the first pressing. This is not quite the same as using a cheese press, but will work quite well if you check the cheese every day and turn it. Be sure to change the cheesecloth, bamboo mat, and board to avoid moisture buildup.

Repeat wrapping and rewrapping the cheese in fresh cheesecloth and pressing it for 1–2 days. Pressing it will encourage moisture loss, which is important if you want a nice firm cheddar. Be sure to change the board each time during the pressing stage.

Allow the cheese to evaporate in the refrigerator (or converted wine fridge) between 40–55°F (4.5–13°C). Evaporation will take up to 5–7 days. (See below for more detail regarding air-drying.)

When the cheese is dry, you can vacuum seal it in plastic bags and continue to age it for 3 months or longer. If you do not vacuum seal it you can then begin the miso brine washing.

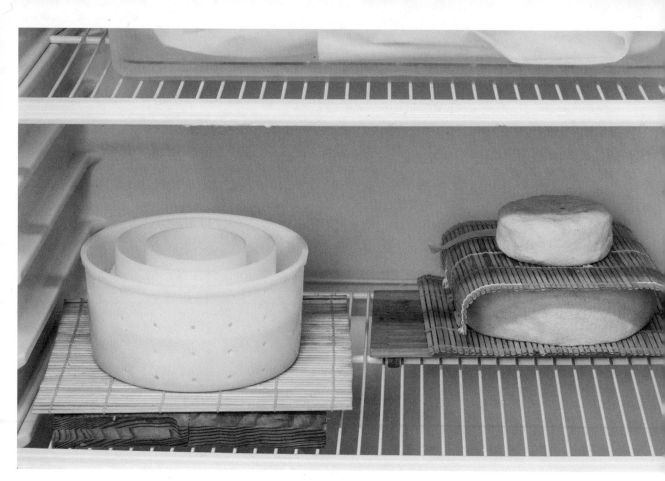

▲ Cheeses aging in a home refrigerator. COLIN MEDHURST

Brine Washing

1. Make brine: For miso brine combine ¼ container of miso — I use chickpea miso — 1 L water, 1 tbsp salt, 1 tbsp white vinegar.
2. If the cheese is quite dry and firm to touch, allow the cheese to soak in the miso brine for up to 3 hours. Remove from brine and allow to air-dry on a sushi mat or board in a cool environment 50°F (10°C) or lower. Turn the cheese 1–2 times a day. Repeat the miso brine washing every 3–4 days after the rind has dried. The brine washing will slow down unwanted growth as well as encourage moisture evaporation and slow down lactic acid production which can lead to bitter flavors if it happens too quickly.

3. If the cheese is very soft, you may also choose to wash the surface with the brine by using cheesecloth soaked in brine and hand washing the surface of the cheese. Dry on bamboo mat as above.

AGING AND RIND CURING METHODS

Within traditional cheesemaking, cheeses are aged and rinds are cured in a number of ways, including rind-washing (including the use of beer and wine on occasion), secondary culture application (mold ripened), and various other methods of working with the microbes to develop flavor and texture. These aging methods are, in part, what determines the naming or classification of the cheeses. In the absence of a formal plant-based cheesemaking classification system, and therefore very much in the spirit of exploration, this section outlines some introductory methods for aging and curing cheese rinds, but does not necessarily try to classify the resulting cheeses. While not exhaustive, the methods below should help you with your plant-based cheesemaking adventure.

Air-Drying

All cheese aging, including for plant-based cheeses, begins with air-drying. Typically, traditional cheeses are aged in "caves," sometimes literally. Most often these days, this aging is done in rooms designed specifically for aging cheeses, allowing temperature and humidity to be controlled, and designed for airflow to circulate in such a way as to encourage evaporation of moisture, a key element of aging.

The two essential environmental variables in aging cheese are temperature and humidity. Ideal cave temperature ranges from 40–55°F (about 4.5–13°C). Humidity requirements depend on the kind of cheese you are making. Since ideal cave conditions are not ideal for refrigeration of other foods, aging cheese at home can be a little trickier.

For home-based cheesemakers, for whom this book is designed, a wine fridge (if you have one you are not using for wine or are inclined to purchase one), can be used, or a cheese-aging box (these can be ordered from cheesemaking supply shops online), in a cool, dry basement or cellar can work. If these are not options for you, and I suspect they are not for most people, then you can do some limited cheese aging in your refrigerator.

For aging in a refrigerator where you are sharing space with other foods, make sure to use a large enough container for your cheese. It is important to make sure that your container will allow for a lot of space around the cheese for good airflow (cheese should only take up 40 percent of space within the container). Place a wood board topped with a bamboo mat in the fridge and rest your cheese on the mat. If the cheese is quite damp, leave it in clean cheesecloth or butter muslin for a couple of days to absorb excess moisture, being sure to flip the cheese daily and change the cheesecloth or butter muslin, if wet. Aging cheese inside a container in the refrigerator will be challenged by the appearance of condensation, a result of the activity of the cultures working. This moisture will have to be wiped away daily, so as to not impede attempts to dry the cheese out. I highly recommend you use butter muslin to wrap the cheese, and change it frequently, if you choose to age cheese inside a container.

Air-drying is essential for evaporation of moisture. As the rind (surface of the cheese) dries, it protects the cheese inside. Excess moisture provides a breeding ground for all yeasts and molds. Most of these are not problematic, especially if the acidity of the cheese is high enough (determined by initial culturing process), and should some grow on your cheese surface, scrape them off and use a heavily salted brine (salt dissolved in water) to wash the surface of the cheese. With respect to so-called wild microbes growing on the surface of your cheese, much will depend on what other food items are in your fridge.

White molds or white fuzz are often wild yeasts and can generally be removed by scraping off the surface and salting or brining the cheese. Grey and black molds are not always or inherently "bad," but, that said, if you do not know what strain they are, and they are growing on your cheeses, it is safest to discard. Blue molds are often related to penicillin and can be removed easily with scraping and salting, but it is not recommended to hold on to the cheese for too long after it first appears. Blue mold spores are readily found on the surface of citrus fruits and if you have some in your fridge it will not be surprising to find your cheeses end up with some blue fuzz periodically. If you find red or pink molds on your cheese, discard it. Many pink molds can produce toxins. Again, without testing to determine the specific strain, it is best to stay safe and discard the cheese.

In general, when making cheese, it is necessary to deep clean your aging and storage unit from time to time to ensure you are removing uninvited molds.

There are some circumstances (bloomy rind cheeses, such as camembert) in which you may want to encourage surface ripening through secondary cultures, but this is a little more challenging to do at home within normal refrigeration methods and while preventing growth of cheese molds on other foods. I do use such methods, and while I don't address them directly in this book, I will be doing so in classes, and in subsequent publications on the development of my processes.

Troubleshooting
Air-Drying at Home

Ensuring that evaporation of moisture occurs evenly will require, as mentioned above, daily flipping and turning of the cheeses. This will also mean changing the bamboo mat, wiping out any excess moisture from the container as whey from the cheese collects, and changing the wood boards that the cheese rests on.

If the cheese dries out too quickly, you will notice cracking of the surface, which means you will need to increase humidity. To increase humidity, you can simply add a clean damp sponge on a plate to your aging container. Cracking of the cheese may also indicate overculturing (too much acidity) which would have occurred in the early culturing process.

Using a hygrometer, which measures both temperature and humidity, is helpful for understanding the aging process of your cheese and how and when to alter conditions by changing temperature or humidity.

Air-drying your cheese will allow you to become very familiar with what to look for during the aging process. Cheeses that have good initial culturing acidity and evaporation of moisture keep longer than moister, less acidic cheeses. To develop other layers of flavor and rind formation, methods such as salt brining and/or rind washing (with or without wine, vinegar, and so on), are used in conjunction with the air-drying process.

Salt Brining and Rind Washing

I use salt brines and other brines to wash rinds in conjunction with air drying. This is a method of curing the rind of semi-soft to hard cheeses to help in removing moisture and controlling the surface growth of airborne molds and bacteria so that the cheeses can continue to age. Cheddar, gouda, and havarti are just some dairy-based cheeses that are salt brined.

In plant-based cheesemaking, you can also salt brine any of the cultured cheeses, provided they are quite firm. This method does not work well with any of the soft cheeses but can be used with semi-hard cheeses when done as a wash versus soaking the cheeses in the brine. That is, you can hand-wash the cheeses with cloth dipped in your brine of choice and wipe down the surface of the cheeses, then allow them to air-dry. Bathing or soaking the semi-hard cheeses will lead to their degradation.

Washing the cheese surface or brining (soaking) the cheeses helps to harden them. Salt leaches moisture from within the cheese, pulling it to the surface, where it then can evaporate or be washed away. This allows the cheese to continue to firm up, and controls surface growth at the same time.

I follow the same approach as dairy cheesemakers in making light, medium, or saturated salt brines.

Light brine 13 oz (approx 370 gm) salt dissolved in 1 gallon (3.78 L) filtered water = 10% salinity.

Medium brine 26 oz (approx 735 gm) salt dissolved in 1 gallon (3.78 L) filtered water = 20% salinity.

Saturated brine 32 oz (approx 907 gm) salt dissolved in 1 gallon (3.78 L) filtered water = 25% salinity (cheese will float in this, if you are doing a soaked brining).

Using Brine

Firm cheeses, such as cultured cheddar or air-dried kefir cheese can be short-soaked in saturated or medium brines. Almond curd that has been significantly air-dried can withstand brine baths quite well. Depending on what I am seeking to achieve or how firm (and salty, because salt will permeate the cheese surface), I will soak cheeses up to 2 days and nights. After removing cheeses from soaking in brine, I will then air-dry them on bamboo mats or cheese-aging mats on top of wooden boards, to allow moisture to be absorbed away from the cheese.

Once the cheese surface has completely dried, I may repeat this process more than once, allowing for drying to occur between soaking. This leads to a very firm surface.

More often than soaking rinds, I usually wash them, using cheesecloth or butter muslin saturated in the brine that I choose, and washing down the sides of the cheese. Again, after washing, I place the cheese on clean bamboo mats or cheese-aging mats to allow them to dry in the refrigerator.

More lightly saturated brines will impart more moisture to the cheese than more heavily saturated brines, so if you do use a lighter brine, be sure to allow the cheese to air-dry fully (as per the directions for air-drying above).

Beer, Wine, Vinegar, or Kombucha Rind Washing

Often, when I want to introduce a different layer of flavor, I will use beer, wine, kombucha, vinegars, or even tea and coffee incorporated into one of the salt brines above to wash the rinds of cheeses. Flavor develops after multiple washing and air-drying cycles. As the moisture evaporates, the flavor of the wine, beer, or other wash permeates the surface of the cheese. I have washed rinds of some cheeses over 2–4 week periods, seeking depth of flavor.

Rind washing in this manner also helps the rind to develop and become quite firm and dry, curing the surface of the cheese.

Cheeses in this book that work well with this kind of treatment are air-dried almond curd, very aged coconut kefir cheese, and the double-cultured cheddar. However, with any of the curds, if you air-dry them long enough for them to become quite firm, you will be able to age them further by washing their rinds.

I often prefer rind washing to bathing, as it does not risk the cheese disintegrating, and you can control the amount of moisture the cheese is absorbing more readily.

Oil Curing

Another method that I sometimes explore in curing my cheese rinds is the use of flavored oils. Herb oils, garlic-infused oil, truffle oil, or smoked oil all offer interesting ways to introduce other flavors into your cheese.

I use butter muslin and wash the rinds in the same manner as I would with a salt brine. I often alternate between using a salt brine, air-drying, then washing with an oil, and again air-drying.

Not to be repetitive, but it is the alternating of the washing process, followed by a drying period, that allows flavor to develop and the cheese rind to firm up.

Dried Herb or Spice Rinds

For cheeses like the coconut kefir cheese, or even any of the other curds that have been drained for a long period of time, and therefore thick enough to work with, you can use dried herbs or spices, mixed with a little salt to cure the rinds.

This is done by simply rubbing them or patting them onto the cheese surface, then setting the cheeses on top of bamboo mats to continue to dry out. It is also necessary to flip and turn the cheeses daily after you apply one of these rind-curing treatments. It is also important to note that dried herbs and spices may carry their own wild yeasts, and these may lead, occasionally, to the blossoming of white spots on the cheese surface, particularly the longer the cheese ages. These are not of concern, and can simply be rubbed or scraped off, and treated with a light salt application.

Dehydrator Use

Very infrequently, I use a dehydrator on lowest temperature setting to assist in removing moisture from a cheese.

If I choose to do this, I use only cheeses that have a high acidity (the cheddar would be a good one), and only for short periods of time, three to six hours. During that time, I flip/turn the cheeses at least once.

I repeat this process every couple of days, and either re-wrap the cheese in cheesecloth/butter muslin, or set it on top of a clean bamboo mat and place it back in the fridge in-between drying sessions.

Bloom Rind Aging

Bloom-ripened or bloomy rind (same thing) cheeses in the dairy world are those such as camembert. "Bloom-ripened cheeses" refers to the use of a culture that is sprayed or washed onto the surface of a cheese (that may or may not be lactic acid cultured first). Using cultures to age cheeses this way is risky in the sense that, as you age them in your refrigerator, the cultures will multiply and can invade other foods.

The cultures commonly used in dairy cheesemaking, and in some of the more advanced plant-based cheeses being explored, commonly involve yeasts and molds such as *Geotrichum*, *Candida*, and *P. camemberti*. They are generally used in specific ratios of yeast/mold together and made into a solution that can be sprayed onto the cheese surface. These ratios will often depend on what flavor and dominant texture a cheesemaker is seeking to achieve.

This is a much more advanced practice, and one I recommend only after you have gained more experience with the other methods first. While this practice is very well established within dairy cheesemaking, even at the level of the home-based cheesemaker, applying this method to plant-based cheeses is still experimental, and not all results or best practices are established formally at this time.

Plant-based cheesemaking is an exciting opportunity to explore self-sustainability, with respect to food production at home, but is, like most good things, one that requires patience and diligence. Do not be disappointed if things do not always turn out the way you hope or imagine, and be prepared to do things more than once.

Be adventurous, be mindful, and be attentive, but have fun, and be open to the prospect of what working with cultured foods can offer you in your culinary adventure.

RESOURCES

DEPENDING ON WHERE you live, you may have more access to materials in your community via health-food and nutrition stores. Additionally, look for homesteading shops and shops catering to those with serious do-it-yourself food impulses. Many of these shops now carry a wide array of specialty process items.

FOOD ITEMS

When and where possible, and within your ability, seek fair trade and organic items.

Cashews, walnuts, sunflower seeds, macadamia nuts, almonds Bulk stores oriented toward healthier, and organic choices will be more likely to have higher quality products. Make sure to smell and feel the nuts. Many nuts and seeds are not stored correctly and are already mildly rancid (that is the oils have begun to leach from them).

Order online from wholesale sources which do not require you to be a commercial business:

- OM Foods: omfoods.com
- The Nut Hut: nuthut.ca

Both are based in British Columbia, but a simple Google search should lead you to suitable suppliers in your area. Even bulk stores should offer reasonable pricing for the home-based experiment.

Coconut milk Look for full fat (low fat will yield lots of whey, but not a lot of kefir or cheese curd). Keep in mind most canned or boxed coconut milk already has water added to it. Look for shops that sell larger cans (more than 500 ml). I find that the larger cans tend to have a better ratio of coconut milk-fat solids to coconut milk water than do the small cans.

Apple cider vinegar This can be found in virtually any grocery store these days. Brands to look for are Omega Nutrition, Braggs, and Spectrum.

Nutritional yeast This can be found in health-food stores, shops focusing on vegan- and vegetarian-friendly markets and, depending on the size of your city, likely even in some of the larger markets such as Whole Foods or even well stocked neighbourhood markets.

Soft wheat berries for making rejuvelac Again, found in health-food or bulk food stores.

Probiotic capsules These are found in any pharmacy, health-food store, or nutrition store.

Look for ones that are in vegetable glycerine capsules *and have not been tested on animals.*

CULTURES
The following cultures and enzymes:

- Coconut kefir or yogurt culture
- Water kefir grains

- Vegetable rennet
- Calcium chloride (can also use pickling calcium chloride,

which is readily available in canning sections of home and hardware stores)

- Cheese cultures (mesophilic direct set)

Can all be ordered online from:
- culturesforhealth.com
- cheesemaking.com
- glengarrycheesemaking.on.ca

EQUIPMENT AND TOOLS

All of the equipment listed below can be found in cookery and culinary supply shops such Ming Wo or Cook Culture (cookculture.com) in British Columbia. But you should be able to find these items readily in many grocery or cooking stores in your location.

- Bamboo/wood cutting boards (for aging cheeses)
- Probe thermometer (digital or otherwise)
- pH meter
- Hygrometer
- Silicone or plastic spoon
- Thick cast (bottom) pots
- Springform pans/ring molds
- Bamboo mats

Most of this equipment can be found in canning supply sections of home and hardware stores.

- Nut milk bags and butter muslin
- Plastic cheese molds
- pH meters and testing kits
- Cheese paper (for wrapping cheeses)

are available from places such as:
- rawnutrition.com
- culturesforhealth.com
- cheesemaking.com
- glengarrycheesemaking.on.ca

It is important to note that nut milk bags are not mandatory. You can make multi-layered cheesecloth or butter muslin bags, but nut milk bags can be re-used.

QUICK REFERENCE GUIDE TO SMELL, TASTE, AND TEXTURE

THIS GUIDE IS primarily to assist you with identifying whether your starter cultures are working and to train you to recognize the range of odor, taste, and texture you can come to expect from a correctly acting culture.

Most of this information is also available at blueheroncheese. com.

CULTURE	SMELL (1–4 DAYS)	SMELL (4–8 DAYS)	TASTE (1–4 DAYS)	TASTE (4–8 DAYS)	TEXTURE (1–4 DAYS)	TEXTURE (4–8 DAYS)
Kefir (on coconut)	Bright Sour	Strong Sour	Mildly sour Yogurt-like	Very sour Tangy Creamish	Smooth Thick Creamy	Starting to firm up into a thick curd/Separation of whey and curd
Kefir (on cashew milk/ paste)	Bright Light sour Nutty Mildly sweet	Strong Sour Nutty Yogurt-like	Mildly sour Yogurt-like Nutty Mildly sweet	Stronger sour flavor Nutty Crème fraîche-like	Thick Creamy Visible activity (bubbles) Expansion of the culturing medium	Thick Creamy Visible activity (bubbles) Some separation of medium and whey
Kefir (on almond milk/ paste)	Fruity (somewhat like frangipane)	Mildly yeasty/ alcohol notes "eggy"	Mildly tangy, fruity, but not sweet Sour, sharp flavor Lightly sulfuric	Sour, sharp flavor Lightly sulfuric	Abundant bubbles Creaminess Some separation of solids from liquid Formation of whey	If highly active, expansion of the kefir, with floating of cream and solids on top of whey
Rejuvelac (on its own)	Lemony or apple cider vinegary	Lightly acidic Fruity Almost like lemonade				
Rejuvelac (coconut)	Yogurt/sour cream-like	Strong Sour cream/ crème fraîche	Tangy Strong Sour cream	Tangy Sour Light nuttiness	Smooth Creamy Thick	Creamy, thick Firm separation of cream solids from whey
Rejuvelac (cashew)	Tangy Sweet Nutty	Stronger sour notes Nutty	Tangy Lightly sweet Mildly nutty	Nutty Yogurt-like Sharper	Thick Creamy Visible bubbles	Very thick separation of whey
Rejuvelac (almond)	Fruity Tangy	Fruity Mild alcohol Sharp	Fruity without sweetness Tangy	Sharp Mildly eggy (due to naturally occurring sulfur compounds)	Thick Creamy Fluffy	Thick Creamy Fluffy Separation of whey

CULTURE	SMELL (1–4 DAYS)	SMELL (4–8 DAYS)	TASTE (1–4 DAYS)	TASTE (4–8 DAYS)	TEXTURE (1–4 DAYS)	TEXTURE (4–8 DAYS)
Probiotic capsule (coconut)	No discernable odor	Mildly yogurt-like	Lightly tangy	Mildly yogurt-like	Kefir-like texture (liquidy)	Lightly thick, but not as thick as other cultures
Probiotic capsule (cashew)	No discernable odor	Lightly tangy notes	Mildly tangy Nutty	Nutty Sour Lightly sweet	Expansion and visible small bubbles Fluffy Effervescent	Visible separation of whey and solids Creamy after drained Chevre-like texture
Probiotic capsule (almond)	Lightly fruity Tangy	Fruity Mildly eggy	Fruity Mildly tangy	Sharp Fruity Mild nut and sulfur notes	Expansion and visible small bubbles	Visible separation of whey and solids Creamy after drained Ricotta-like texture

ABOUT THE AUTHOR

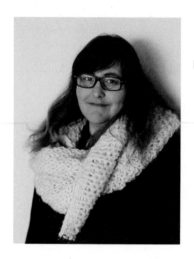

A **BORN AND BRED** west coaster from Alert Bay, BC, Chef Karen McAthy has worked in and around kitchens since 2000. Her interest in and passion for local food systems and growing food was well established in her previous posts as director of food services at W2 Media Arts, executive chef of Graze Vegetarian (now closed), and Zend Conscious Lounge. Karen left Zend in July 2016 to pursue plant-based cheese making, catering, and teaching classes with her company, Blue Heron Creamery. A published author, Karen's first book, *The Art of Plantbased Cheesemaking* was published with New Society Publishers, spring 2017.

With both parents coming from agricultural backgrounds, Karen grew up learning how to grow food, and being curious about the wild plants in the woods of her home island. A deep desire to learn and understand how things work informs Karen's pursuit of making plantbased food and her ongoing interest in culturing processes. Her academic background in political science and biology finds itself present in her daily work as a chef as she brings a focus on the various ecological and ethical issues readily present in the food industry.

Karen can be contacted at chef@blueheroncheese.com

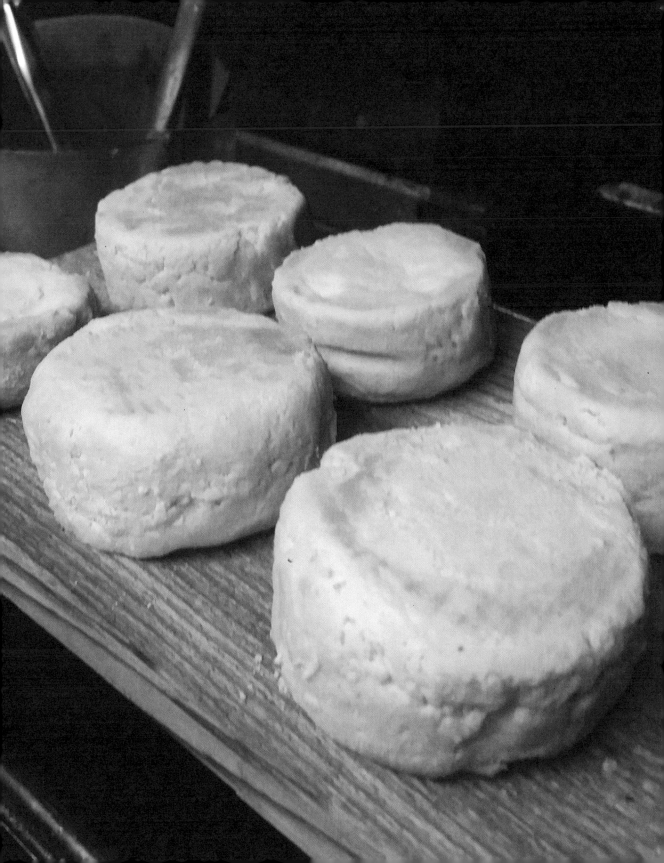

ABOUT NEW SOCIETY PUBLISHERS

New Society Publishers is an activist, solutions-oriented publisher focused on publishing books for a world of change. Our books offer tips, tools, and insights from leading experts in sustainable building, homesteading, climate change, environment, conscientious commerce, renewable energy, and more — positive solutions for troubled times.

We're proud to hold to the highest environmental and social standards of any publisher in North America. This is why some of our books might cost a little more. We think it's worth it!

▶ We print all our books in North America, never overseas

▶ All our books are printed on **100% post-consumer recycled paper**, processed chlorine-free, with low-VOC vegetable-based inks (since 2002)

▶ Our corporate structure is an innovative employee shareholder agreement, so we're one-third employee-owned (since 2015)

▶ We're carbon-neutral (since 2006)

▶ We're certified as a B Corporation (since 2016)

At New Society Publishers, we care deeply about *what* we publish — but also about *how* we do business.

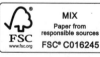
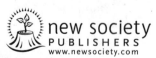

new society
PUBLISHERS
www.newsociety.com

New Society Publishers
ENVIRONMENTAL BENEFITS STATEMENT

For every 5,000 books printed, New Society saves the following resources:[1]

30	Trees
2,695	Pounds of Solid Waste
2,965	Gallons of Water
3,867	Kilowatt Hours of Electricity
4,899	Pounds of Greenhouse Gases
12	Pounds of HAPs, VOCs, and AOX Combined
7	Cubic Yards of Landfill Space

[1]Environmental benefits are calculated based on research done by the Environmental Defense Fund and other members of the Paper Task Force who study the environmental impacts of the paper industry.